WEIGHT, SEX, AND MARRIAGE

Weight, Sex, and Marriage

A Delicate Balance

❦❖❦

RICHARD B. STUART

AND

BARBARA JACOBSON

W · W · NORTON & COMPANY

New York · London

Published simultaneously in Canada by Penguin Books Canada Ltd.,
2801 John Street, Markham, Ontario L3R 1B4.
Printed in the United States of America.

The text of this book is composed in Bembo, with
display type set in Bembo. Composition and
manufacturing by The Haddon Craftsmen, Inc.
Book design by Jacques Chazaud.

Library of Congress Cataloging-in-Publication Data

Stuart, Richard B.
Weight, sex, and marriage.

Bibliography: p.
Includes index.
1. Obesity—Psychological aspects. 2. Obesity—
Social aspects. 3. Sex in marriage. 4. Body weight.
I. Jacobson, Barbara. II. Title.
RC552.02S78 1987 616.3'98'0019 86–33148

ISBN 0-393-02466-0

W. W. Norton & Company, Inc., 500 Fifth Avenue, New York, N. Y. 10110
W. W. Norton & Company Ltd., 37 Great Russell Street, London WC1B 3NU

2 3 4 5 6 7 8 9 0

Contents

Authors' Note

The heart of this book comes from the thousands of women who have shared their private and often painful secrets with us. We thank them for their candor, and assure them that all identifying details of the stories we recount have been altered in order to respect their privacy.

WEIGHT, SEX, AND MARRIAGE

I

Looking for Answers:
Our Own Experience

We have a personal attachment to the subject of this book, because it was our mutual interest in weight control that led us to meet, and eventually marry. Fifteen years ago, Richard, though not overweight, was professionally committed to finding the elusive secret of successful weight loss. Barbara, who was overweight, was personally committed to the same quest.

Richard's interest in weight control began in 1965, when a woman named Elaine came to him for psychotherapy. She was in her mid-thirties, and about sixty pounds overweight. Although she considered herself a good mother, a loving wife, and a competent executive secretary, Elaine was convinced that she was a failure as a person. The telltale proof: a lifetime of dieting failures.

Elaine started at least five diets every year. With the best of the diets, she lost less than ten pounds, and she regained the weight as quickly as it was lost. And with each unsuccessful effort, she added a few extra pounds, and lost a bit more self-confidence.

Past attempts at psychotherapy hadn't been very helpful. Two years of analysis helped her gain insight into the childhood experiences that contributed to her weight problem. Unfortunately, insight wasn't all she gained; she ended therapy fourteen pounds heavier than she had been at the start!

With each setback, Elaine became more obsessed with her weight. Eventually, weight concerns completely dominated her thoughts. She explored the most extreme weight loss methods available. First she considered being one of the first patients to have her jaws wired, but decided this would only add to her flawed appearance. She inquired about intestinal bypass surgery, but felt the risks would be too great. She even considered shock therapy, but couldn't find a physician who would go to that extreme to help her control her weight-related depression. When she was about to hit bottom, she called Richard, and implored him to free her from the tyranny of her obsession with food.

Richard doubted he could help. He told Elaine that she'd already received the most common psychological treatment for obesity, and it obviously hadn't helped. But Elaine was insistent, hinting that she'd rather be dead than fat.

Richard agreed to accept her as a patient, but said he'd need a few weeks to do some library research. Unfortunately, long hours in the library only increased his sense of futility. The professional literature was rife with speculations and contradictions. Some writers described obesity as a defense against pregnancy but other believed it to be a symbolic pregnancy. Some researchers saw fat as a rejection of femininity in which the obese woman avoids living up to the feminine ideal. Yet it was also seen as a rejection of masculinity in which the overweight woman accentuates all the features of the female persona.

These Freudian paradoxes were not only confusing, they were also unfounded. Little or no evidence supported their truth, nor was there any proof that the insights, even if they were valid, could lead to successful weight loss.

Going beyond the psychoanalytic view, Richard still found

little cause for optimism. Nutritionists believed that people were overweight because they didn't know how to eat properly. Yet their own studies indicated that obese women usually knew more about nutrition than most of the doctors who treated them. Psychologists described the problem in terms of a lack of will-power or self-control, but no existing therapeutic techniques were effective in strengthening those weaknesses. Exercise specialists attributed obesity to laziness, but they had few suggestions about how to make exercise appealing. And physicians bemoaned the obese patient's lack of motivation, yet were at a loss as to how to inspire their patients to start losing weight.

It was clear that the professional view of overweight people was judgmental, harsh, and distressingly bleak. Obesity was generally seen as a psychological disease for which there was no cure.

But there was one hopeful theoretical perspective suggesting that behavioral self-management might be useful in treating obesity. Richard told Elaine he couldn't offer her a well-tested therapy, but he would be willing to experiment with a new approach if she wanted to take that risk. Eager to try anything, Elaine enthusiastically agreed.

Fifty-two weeks later, and forty-five pounds lighter, Elaine referred three friends with weight problems, and in time they matched her success. Within two years, Richard's clients were almost exclusively overweight women, many of whom were finally able to meet their weight loss goals.

Richard reported these results in professional journals, and published his techniques in a book, *Slim Chance In A Fat World*. Soon after that, he started to work with Weight Watchers International. This gave him the opportunity to offer behavioral techniques to hundreds of thousands of people, while continuing to search for even more effective methods.

Around this time, Barbara volunteered to help Richard with his research. Although she said that her interest was simply academic, she was privately hoping to be among the first to benefit from any new weight-control discoveries.

Barbara had started her training as a "professional dieter" while still in high school and at a normal weight. Driven by the desire to be as thin as the models in the teen magazines, she tried one fad diet after another. Soon she was trapped in the endless cycle of semi-starvation and binge eating.

What started out as an imaginary weight problem developed into a real one by the time Barbara finished her first year of college. By then she was virtually majoring in dieting, and she studied the intricacies of the popular diets with a dedication that other students reserved for the final in Great Books 101.

In addition to the old standbys like Stillman and Atkins, she tried diets of her own invention, such as the "yogurt only" diet and the "500-calories-a-day" plan. She also tried over-the-counter diet pills, diet doctors, fasting, and anything else that offered the hope of eliminating unwanted pounds. Nothing worked for long. The only result of these dieting attempts was an ever increasing obsession with food and weight. Her body stubbornly maintained itself even while she starved, and weight loss seemed an impossible dream.

Barbara decided to dedicate herself to the study of obesity, and so began our collaboration. We started by exploring the effectiveness of the current weight-loss treatments. While behavior modification programs were more successful than any other, they seldom produced substantial weight losses that could be maintained. Behavior modification clearly wasn't a complete solution.

And so we returned to the professional literature in search of new discoveries. We were especially interested to see if there might be an "obese personality" that could explain why some people struggled with weight problems while others stayed thin, seemingly without effort. But no answers were forthcoming. All we learned was that there were so many overweight people, with such varied life experiences, that it was absurd even to think that they might all have the same personality traits.

Once we acknowledged that research wasn't going to provide answers, we decided to take a more personal approach. We interviewed overweight women to see how they viewed their own eating problems. These women helped us understand that the trigger for overeating was seldom simply a "loss of willpower." Instead, the culprit seemed to be the stress of daily life which led to negative feelings that they could pacify only by over-eating.

As we changed our focus from food to feelings, we found increasing evidence that most overeating was indeed a response to boredom, loneliness, anger, anxiety, or depression. For many people, these moods had to be brought under control before new eating patterns could be developed and maintained. Armed with this new insight, Richard wrote *Act Thin, Stay Thin,* which offered a menu of techniques for both weight and mood control.

This combination seemed to improve weight-loss results, but maintenance was still a major problem, especially for women who had lost many pounds. As soon as the novelty of weight loss wore off, these women reverted to the familiar old patterns of overeating. Letters like the following were common:

> Dear Dr. Stuart:
>
> I've learned how to manage my eating well enough to reach my goal weight. But I just can't diet forever. If I lose 30 pounds, I keep the weight off for six months, and then regain 35. I consider myself a successful dieter—yet I'm heavier now than when I first set out to reach my goal!
>
> I know my problem isn't biological, because I've proven I can lose. So I'm afraid it must be psychological. Where do I go next?
>
> Sincerely,
> A Yo-yo Whose String Is Wearing Thin

Letters like this were puzzling. The women who wrote them were all involved in a well-designed weight program. They had lost weight at a medically acceptable rate. They learned to manage their moods. They became skilled in eating management techniques. They learned to follow a prudent diet. And still they regained the weight they'd worked so hard to lose. What was left to change?

Again we turned to interviews, this time focusing on women who had lost and then regained at least 100 pounds. Much to our surprise, not one of these women was baffled by her failure to maintain goal weight. Each could pinpoint a moment when she thought something like: "Staying thin just isn't worth the effort! I think I'll eat a chocolate cake."

We were even more startled to learn that most of these women didn't regain their weight because they found *eating* irresistible; they were drawn by the *appeal of being fat*. Being thin created problems that weight gain would at least temporarily solve.

An insight from an unexpected source helped us realize one of the common ways in which a woman's fat could be of use. Richard was treating a woman who was not obese, but alcoholic. After ten years of drinking, she had successfully completed a treatment program and was thrilled with her accomplishment. She naturally expected her husband to praise her efforts and be delighted with her success. Instead, he did everything he could to end her sobriety. He tempted her with alcohol. He increased his own drinking. He started finding fault with almost everything she did. And when all his pressure failed to drive her to drink, he filed for divorce.

Her story revealed an unsettling truth: personal problems often play a role in keeping relationships stable. For some reason, this woman's husband was only comfortable when she had a drinking problem. As the story unfolded, it became clear that the husband had a very low opinion of himself. In retrospect, it appeared that his wife's alcoholism allowed him to feel equal in a relationship that was otherwise quite threatening to him. After she overcame her major weakness, he could not tolerate the shift in power. When he couldn't pull her back down to his level, he left the marriage.

This woman wanted to stay married, but recognized her dilemma. She felt certain her husband would come back . . . if she started drinking again. But because she was determined never to allow herself to become dependent on alcohol again, she turned to therapy for help.

This woman's story painfully illustrated the intimate relationship between marital and individual problems. Marital distress may have contributed to her drinking, but her alcoholism also helped stabilize her marriage.

This led us to wonder if it was possible that a wife's obesity might have a similar function in other marriages. It was time to examine the ways in which overeating and marriage might interact. Perhaps an understanding of this relationship would provide another missing piece in the puzzle.

To continue our search for answers, we published a questionnaire in a national magazine directed toward weight-conscious women. Fifteen thousand women responded, and many enclosed letters describing the intricate connections between weight and marriage. Because sexual concerns were so frequently mentioned, we followed up the original survey with a second one focusing on weight and sex. This time 9,000 women responded, and once again many shared personal stories ranging from a few sentences to eleven single spaced typed pages. (Of these, only four criticized us for "prying" into their private lives!)

The letters came from teenagers and grandmothers, from housewives and career women, and from women in first, second, and third marriages. Some of the respondents had successfully maintained their goal weight for years, while others were still desperately searching for ways to lose 100 pounds or more.

Our average respondent was a woman in her mid-thirties, who had completed some college, and worked at least half-time outside her home. She was in her first marriage, was the mother of two children, and had an annual family income of approximately $35,000.

Because our sample represents a reasonable cross-section of weight-conscious American women, we can make some observations about the powerful strains that result when weight problems are intertwined with sexual and marital concerns. Thanks to what we learned from our respondents, we're closer to understanding why so many women have trouble losing weight. They put too much emphasis on restricting food intake, and give too little consideration to *why* they overeat.

The "why" of overeating is crucial. A woman's weight problem is not isolated from the rest of her life. Weight and body image are in delicate balance with her marital happiness, sexual satisfaction, and self-esteem. It's important to understand not only how weight change affects these other aspects of a woman's life, but also how life problems influence her weight. Until these relationships are understood, she is likely to be baffled and frustrated by repeated weight-loss failures.

In the following chapters, we'll explore these complex relationships. First we'll focus on women who want to be thin, but need to overeat to relieve emotional strain and sexual frustration. Then we'll look at women who believe their extra weight keeps their marriages stable. Some intentionally stay overweight, while others feel victimized by husbands who have their own reasons for wanting fat wives. We'll describe the astonishing variety of benefits that both husbands and wives derive from a wife's weight problems. Understanding these benefits will help clarify the ambivalence many women have about being thin.

We believe that overeating and becoming overweight are

understandable responses to life stresses, but they're seldom the best, and they're *never* the only choices women can make. By uncovering the deeper functions of food and fat, it's easier to make a realistic assessment of the costs and benefits of losing weight. Then women can evaluate how the decision to lose (or not to lose) might influence their lives and their marriages.

For those who do decide that weight loss is worth the effort, we'll outline our "indirect" approach to weight management. Traditional weight-control programs generally use the "direct" approach by focusing on resisting the temptation to eat. In effect, the direct approach tells women: "Try to forget about *why* you overeat, and follow our guidelines for *what* and *how* and *when* to eat."

Unfortunately, ignoring the reasons for overeating doesn't make the reasons disappear, and eventually they can sabotage even the most well-designed diet. So we offer a different message: "You may have some good reasons for overeating. Let's try to understand those reasons, so you can change some of the situations and feelings that lead you to overeat."

Once those changes are made, we help women develop a personalized, permanent weight-control program. Here, too, our approach is different. Rather than recommending steady rapid weight loss until goal weight is achieved, we suggest *gradual* weight loss with some "rest stops" along the way. This allows the body and mind to adjust to the changes caused by losing weight. And instead of insisting on a specific diet, we suggest the use of a *self-selected eating plan* that allows each woman to continue to eat many of the foods she most enjoys. We'll offer guidelines for creating a plan, but each woman will then develop the details that are most relevant to herself and her way of life.

Finally, we offer married women guidelines for deciding what role they want their husbands to play. Since husbands can do a great deal to help or hinder weight-loss efforts, we suggest that women discuss their plans with their husbands, and *ask for the kind of help they want.*

Our book would not have been possible without the survey respondents, clients, interested volunteers, and Weight Watchers members who took the time to share intimate details of their private lives with us. We are deeply grateful to them.

Some of these women thanked us, for helping them discuss these personal matters for the first time in their lives. They had spent years worrying about their weight, but had never considered the marital and sexual aspects of their weight problems. As they started to unravel these tangled relationships, they felt less overwhelmed, and more able to confront their problems directly.

By taking the personal meanings of food and fat "out of the closet," we hope that every woman with a similar problem will realize she is not alone. By explaining the "indirect" approach to weight loss, we hope to convince any woman who is overwhelmed by her weight problem that she need not feel helpless or hopeless. By recognizing and changing the *reasons* for overeating, a woman can not only lose weight, but she can also greatly improve the quality of her life.

II

The Many Uses of Food
in Marriage

Judy came to us for weight loss treatment the week after her thirty-seventh birthday. This was a particularly depressing time for her; not only was she still single, but she was as many pounds overweight as she was years old. Judy ignored her weight for years, believing that if she found someone to marry, her extra weight would naturally disappear. She reasoned that marriage would end her loneliness and depression, thereby ending her need to console herself with food.

Anna, another of our clients, is the same age and weight as Judy. But she's the married mother of three. Her weight problem began with the birth of her first child, and weight has been a concern ever since. Anna confesses that sometimes she longs for the freedom of the single life. Without her husband, children, house, and dog to look after, she's sure she'd have more time and energy to attend to her own needs, including her need to lose weight.

Nowhere is the "grass is always greener" phenomenon better illustrated than in the envy that exists between married and single women. Of course, each situation has its pleasures and problems. But when it comes to weight problems, married women seem to have more than their share. Indeed, weight gain after marriage is so common for both women and men that it's rare to find a couple who can fit into their honeymoon outfits on their fifth anniversary. One woman who gained twenty-five pounds in her first two years of marriage wistfully commented that the surgeon general should stamp marriage licenses with the warning: "Marriage is hazardous to your weight."

Of course, marriage isn't the only culprit, but it does speed the leap into larger sizes . . . at least according to our survey respondents. During 13 years of marriage, the average woman gained 24.7 pounds, while her husband gained 19.4.

The letters we received offered many explanations for weight gain during marriage. Sometimes women relax and stop worrying about keeping their weight down once they enjoy and trust the security of marriage. More often, the responsibilities and stresses of being a wife and mother lead women down the aisle to the half-size department. Finally, some women live with marital and sexual problems that make overeating feel like the key to emotional survival. We'll examine all of these situations as we pinpoint forces that make weight gain such a common part of married life.

A LICENSE TO RELAX

Marriage is full of surprises . . . not all of them pleasing. The niceties of courtship are usually abandoned by the end of the honeymoon, and newlyweds learn all too quickly what "real life" will be like. Whether marriage turns out to be a joy or a disappointment, one thing is virtually certain: married life will bear little resemblance to the idyllic days of courtship. For marriage is a game played by an entirely different set of rules.

We're on our very best behavior during courtship. Our goal

is not to tell the truth, the whole truth, and nothing but the truth: it's to win the dating game.

Courtship is the time of maximum human deception. Never do we work as hard to present ourselves in such a positive light. In trying to get to "I do," both men and women set aside their own wants and needs, and dedicate themselves to pleasing the object of their affections.

But marriage changes all that. Perhaps it's due to the belief that marriage is "forever." Divorce statistics aside, everyone enters marriage with the conviction that the union will last a lifetime. This expectation has profound effects: while it may have been easy to be on one's best behavior for a short time, no one expects to keep up the act for a lifetime.

In addition, a marriage license is like a diploma—it's a sign that crucial tests have been passed. Spouses are no more likely to keep trying to qualify for their license than students are to retake courses they've already passed. Instead, most of the effort put into pleasing each other is diverted to work, home, and eventually children.

The demise of courtship can start a woman's drift toward post-marital weight problems. Secure in her husband's acceptance, and the legal bonds of marriage, a wife may feel less concerned about her weight. Freed from the need to compete in the singles market, and only too happy to give up the stress and strain of dieting, she may see marriage as the chance to end years of self-denial.

Laura, a woman in her late twenties, had been married five years when she started to worry about the twenty-three pounds she'd gained:

> Before I got married, crash diets were as much a part of my life as work and sleep. For five days a week I'd starve, in order to be able to eat all I wanted on weekend

dates. Looking my best was my top priority, and I didn't mind doing what it took to look good in tight jeans or a slinky evening dress.

But once I settled into married life, I lost all my willpower. I think it was because I knew my husband loved me and would stay with me no matter how I looked. There just wasn't any point in continuing to put myself through the agonies of dieting. So now I eat what I want, and I feel much less deprived. But since I've decided to let myself go, I've gone up three dress sizes.

Laura went on to explain her feeling that food did *not* serve an important psychological function for her. She was happily married and thoroughly enjoyed her job. Because she was content most of the time, she didn't think she used food as an emotional crutch. She didn't binge or feel obsessed with weight. She just consumed more calories than she used, and the difference was large enough for her to gain three to five pounds a year. She wanted to lose weight, but felt her self-worth wasn't dependent on the number on the scale. The trouble was, at the rate Laura was gaining, in another five years she might weigh 50 to 60 pounds more than when she married.

Many of the wives who gradually gain weight are joined by their husbands. Enjoying food together is a pleasure neither spouse wants to curtail, but eventually the effects can't be ignored:

Our marriage is so comfortable for us that we've lost the trim figures we once had. It took only two years to put extra weight on, slowly but surely. Dieting is hard for us, because we don't see ourselves as fat. Yet our clothes are becoming tighter and tighter. If we don't do something, we'll soon be crossing the barrier from "pleasingly" to "not-so-pleasingly" plump!

The fact that weight gain is gradual and eating patterns are normal doesn't mean that weight loss will be easy. The biggest challenge these women face is finding the motivation to start and stick to a weight-loss plan.

When life is going smoothly, and weight doesn't interfere with feelings of self-worth, it's hard to find the inspiration to change. Especially when the only perceived alternative to weight gain is stringent dieting, it's easy to put off dieting until tomorrow—or forever—while enjoying the pleasures of today.

THE MOST FATTENING JOB IN THE WORLD

If we were asked to design the most fattening job in the world, what would the job description include?

We'd start with a work setting that allowed easy access to a wide variety of foods. We'd insist that the worker take responsibility for planning meals, shopping, cooking, and cleaning up, so as to keep attention constantly focused on food and eating. And we'd add enough mundane tasks to create a level of boredom that makes eating seem interesting in comparison.

Working hours would begin early in the morning and continue until late at night. This would encourage the worker to replenish waning energy with extra nourishment. And the job should involve minimal contact with adults. Isolating the worker would make it easier to stop caring about physical appearance, and the loneliness would make food an enticing companion.

Finally, the job should be low on the status scale, in order to suppress the worker's self-esteem. Lack of status could be achieved by making it a volunteer effort, since job status is usually evaluated by salary. Having no income, the worker would have to be financially dependent upon someone else, and would have to accept the lack of power that accompanies this dependence.

What we call the job is unimportant. Whether the label is "housewife," "full-time mother," "homemaker," or even "domestic engineer," the problems remain the same. Any woman who chooses to stay home full-time to take care of the house and children will confront the stresses of this potentially fattening job.

In all the discussions of the costs and benefits of this traditional woman's role, we seldom see reference to its relationship to obesity. Yet from our earliest research on weight problems, we found that a major predictor of a woman's success is whether or not she works outside her home.[1] Women who don't hold outside jobs consistently have a very hard time losing weight. The reasons are obvious from the job description!

Although neither of our recent weight surveys inquired about the role of the housewife/mother, many women fitting that description revealed how their daily routines influenced their weight. Most felt driven to cope with stress, fatigue, and boredom by escaping to the kitchen for some edible relief.

We found that the younger mothers were hardest on themselves. The swift move from teenager to bride to mother often left them inundated with responsibilities and confused by their dissatisfaction. They believed they should be happy and fulfilled, but instead felt empty and depressed.

A young mother named Mary was 25 pounds overweight and severely depressed when she came to us for help. This is how she first described her problem:

> I have two beautiful children and a hard-working husband. That makes me luckier than a lot of women. But for some reason, I'm always depressed. Only food cheers me up, though never for very long. I know I have to stop this crazy eating and start losing weight, but it's hard to stick to a diet when I'm depressed. I don't know what's wrong with me, but I know I need help!

The more we learned about Mary's life, the better we understood her depression. She was very lonely growing up, and she had always looked forward to having a family of her own. She married her high school sweetheart the week after graduation, and was pregnant when they returned from their honeymoon. By her twenty-second birthday, she had twin three-year-old sons and a life that didn't come close to her fantasies of familial bliss.

Mary's first disappointment was her discovery that her husband wasn't much interested in being a father. He worked long hours selling insurance, and when he was home, he wanted to settle down with a beer and the television. Mary appreciated her husband's dedication to his work and his ability to earn a good living. She didn't mind the long hours, but she was lonely even when he was home.

Mary also hadn't realized how much work was involved in being a mother. She had dreamed of summer afternoons at the playground in the park, and joyful little faces on Christmas morning. But the reality consisted of gray winter days trapped in the house with whining, bored children and mounting piles of dirty laundry. Her few opportunities to get out of the house were usually limited to errands, or to chauffeuring her children to friends' houses or the pediatrician.

Eating was one of Mary's few available pleasures. In fact, she believed that eating kept her sane. It provided distraction when her patience was wearing thin, entertainment when she was overcome with boredom, and comfort when she needed it:

> I need food to help me cope. There's so much to do every day, and I get really flustered when the children's demands prevent me from making any progress on my chores. I start to feel overwhelmed, and I get down on myself . . . trying to figure out "What am I doing wrong? How am I wasting time?" That's when I start to get

angry at the kids. I love them so much, but I'm afraid that if I couldn't control myself by eating, I'd end up losing my temper and hurting one of them. Maybe that's why there's hardly a time during the day when I don't have something in my mouth.

Sometimes, when I realize that I'm feeling angry at these innocent little children, I think I'm a horrible, selfish person. Then I get even more depressed, and eat even more to try to blot out the bad feelings. I don't know how to break out of this cycle of frustration, depression, and binge eating.

Like so many other women, Mary kept her frustration to herself, assuming that she was the only mother who had trouble coping. Concluding that her personal flaws were the cause of her suffering, she felt helpless and worthless. The more her self-esteem plummeted, the more she turned to food for consolation.

Mary's self-blame was partly the result of having become a mother while she was still in her teens. She had never held a job, and she had few experiences with which to compare her current situation. In her first attempt to live as an adult, she felt she had failed.

Women who were employed before making the decision to stay home with their children often have a clearer understanding of the challenges of being a full-time housewife and mother. They realize that circumstances, not personality deficits, are at least partially responsible for their weight gain.

Many of our survey respondents reported that they never had a weight problem until they became full-time, stay-at-home mothers. One woman presented a long list of things that had contributed to a 33 pound weight gain over the two years since she had quit her job. In her opinion, the most important was the lack of adult companionship. She didn't miss her job per se, but she longed for the conversations with co-workers that enlivened every day. Without this vital contact, eating become her only distraction.

Other women believed that not having daily contact with men diminished their motivation to look their best: "When I had a regular job, I keep my weight down because I know the men at work would notice. But now that I'm not working, I'm rarely seen except at the grocery store, so why worry about 20 or 30 extra pounds?"

Fatigue can also take its toll. Especially when women are caring for parents as well as husbands and children, the demands can become oppressive:

> I have three children from my previous marriage, and one with my husband. We also have joint custody of my husband's two teenagers, who spend more time with us every year. I also care for my father who is 89, senile, and demands as much attention as a baby. Taking care of all these people plus my husband is more work than two full-time jobs. But I also try to help out financially by selling newspaper subscriptions by phone. I wake up at 6:15 every day, I'm on the run till 10 at night, and I'm constantly exhausted. The only—and I mean ONLY—thing I get to do for myself is eat.

This woman has become a professional nurturer. She spends almost every waking moment caring for other people, and gets little attention and comfort in return. When she naturally runs out of steam and is feeling drained, she seeks a quick fix in kitchen.

Although many housewives are overworked, lonely, and constantly tired, the most common complaint is boredom. This was a particularly dominant theme in the letters from rural women.

Many described their lives in ways that dispel city-dwellers' myths about country living. They painted pictures of a hard and lonely existence in which eating is not just the best, but the *only* diversion from monotony:

> I am a rancher's wife and the mother of two little boys. Since I live 12 miles from the closest town, I don't get to see people often. And even when we do go out, all we do is eat. What else can you do in a town of 700 people? There was a bowling alley 30 miles away, but it burned down. And the only movie theater within an hour's drive has no heat, so we can only go in the summer. I like to sew and watch TV, but I still get bored a lot, especially during those long dark winter months. If I couldn't entertain myself by eating, I think I'd go berserk.

Still, one doesn't have to live in the country to be bored. Of all the letters from unhappy housewives, one of the saddest came from a suburban woman who was struggling to compensate for the sacrifices she felt she made when she chose to become a full-time mother:

> From 6:30 in the morning until late at night when I put away the toys, I do chores that bore me, play games that don't interest me, and have dull, redundant, conversations with my children. Even when I see other women, all we do is talk about our children . . . what else happens in our lives? All I do for pleasure is eat, and I realize even that bores me. My life is so empty that I pray I'll wake up and find my youngest child in school so I'll be free to spend at least part of my waking life as a *person* instead of just a mother.

Of course, this excerpt represents an extreme. But it illustrates the important point that housewife/mothers can feel engulfed by their job responsibilities. Despite the rewards of caring for children—and there are many—the life of a professional nurturer can be very draining. Mothers of young children constantly give their energy, their patience, their attention, and their labor, with few opportunities to replenish their diminishing reserves.

While there are other ways to deal with the stresses of the wife/mother job, eating often turns out to be the easiest temporary solution. Food is always available, it offers immediate satisfaction, and it can be consumed while caring for a house and children. But overeating provides a short-term "time-out" with long-term consequences.

The obesity that results from tranquilizing unhappiness with food can't help but add stress in the long run. Excess weight compounds feelings of depression and nibbles away at a woman's self-confidence. Chronic feelings of depression and worthlessness can keep a woman at home even after her children are older and out of the house all day. So what begins as a temporary respite from loneliness, fatigue, and boredom builds a wall of self-consciousness that further traps a woman in the situation that made her so unhappy in the first place.

STARVING FOR LOVE

Recently we heard several women discussing a columnist's belief that not getting enough hugs can cause depression.

"So now it's been proved that everybody needs hugs!" one woman exclaimed. To which another added, "If you can't get a hug, a chocolate bar will do!"

We smiled at her confirmation of a conviction many people have held for years. The unsatisfied hunger for touch is mysteriously transformed into hunger for food. But carrots and broccoli won't do. For the touch-deprived, only sweets hold that special magic normally found in a tender embrace. What vitamin pills offer to those who don't have adequate nutrition, sweets provide for the emotionally malnourished.

Food becomes associated with love early in life. An anxious infant is comforted with milk. Baby's first words and steps are often rewarded with sweets. Lollipops may be used to distract young children from the pain of shots at the doctor's office. And ice cream, cake, and other edible delights are the hallmarks of birthdays, holidays, and an array of other happy occasions. It's not surprising that when our attempts to find comfort, support, and love are unsuccessful, we habitually turn to favored foods to satisfy our psychological needs.

Of all appealing foods, chocolate enjoys top billing. Some scientists believe that chocolate contains a chemical similar to the substance that naturally occurs in our bodies when we're on a "romantic high." If true, this would explain why so many women crave chocolate when they feel the need for love and affection.

For its apostles, chocolate provides a semi-spiritual experience that makes life worth living:

> Chocolate can do wonderful things for your overall sense of well-being. It can offset disappointments, allay frustrations, provide joy and comfort—even inspire romance.[2]

> Brownies are high on the list of security foods. A generous bite of brownie, lavished with nuts or frosting, is uniquely satisfying, an experience that renews faith in life's goodness despite hard times or personal disappointment.[3]

After all, when you get right down to it, having one of our mouth-watering brownies around is a matter of survival.[4]

Another tribute to the popularity of chocolate is the profusion of books and magazines devoted entirely to chocolate. Some, of course, focus on recipes, but others delve into chocolate lore, chocolate fantasies, and chocolate addiction. Titles include phrases like "quick fix," "kisses," and "seduction." This connection between sweet eating and sensual pleasure is further emphasized by the women who refer, only semi-jokingly, to "eating orgasms" as they describe the highs of enjoying their favorite foods.

The ability to attain this kind of sensual high is particularly convenient when eating is a woman's only reliable source of pleasure. When her marriage lacks the sexual and affectionate expressiveness she craves, she can turn to food for love. Since almost one-third of the women in our survey reported being less than satisfied with their sex lives, we assume that many thousands —possibly millions—may turn to food when love and affection are scarce.

As in most other studies, women in our survey reported having intercourse with their husbands approximately eight times per month. Not surprisingly, the happily married had intercourse 10.3 times per month, while those in unhappy marriages had sex less than half as often.

It's impossible to tell from the survey results whether a good marriage leads to more frequent sex, or whether sexual frequency makes a marriage happier. But other researchers found that when the nonsexual part of a couple's life is going badly, their sex life also suffers.[5] And based on our clinical experience, we're convinced that happy marriages predict happy sex lives, rather than the other way around. While all happily married women may not be sexually satisfied, women with good sex lives are also likely to be happy with their marriages.

Of course an active sex life doesn't always mean a happy one. A few women in our survey wished that their husbands had *less* sexual interest. For example:

> We make love 15–20 times a month and it's not enough for him. He'd do it EVERY DAY if I let him, he's that much of a maniac about sex. I just wish he'd be like other men and be happy with once a week! I was brought up believing that sex is something special that you shouldn't do all the time. For me, routine sex is worse than no sex at all.

However, comments like these were extremely rare. The vast majority of women who were unhappy with the frequency of sex wanted intercourse *more* often than their husbands did. They were particularly frustrated when the number of times fell to less than once a week.

We found a range of situations involving wives who wanted more sexual contact than their husbands did. Stereotypes aside, some men simply aren't interested in sex. If the marriage is good in other respects, their wives will find ways to adjust to the lack of physical intimacy. As one woman wrote:

> My husband isn't a sexual person. We weren't even sexually active on our honeymoon, and since then, he's been satisfied to have no sex at all. Fortunately, he's very kind, and our marriage is good in every other way, so I've learned to live with no sex, even though I miss it terribly. When I feel sexually frustrated, I usually turn to my favorite foods.

There are many potential explanations for a man's disinterest in sex. It could be the result of hormonal problems, aging, miseducation about sex, a bad marriage, fatigue, or preoccupation with other concerns. It can also be a symptom of physical or emotional illness. Whatever the cause, many husbands will not seek help, forcing wives to cope with frustration:

> Our sexual problems started when my husband be-
> came impotent. I've begged him to get help, but he's too
> embarrassed to tell anyone. He'd rather just live without
> sex, and he's started to treat me like I'm his roommate
> instead of his wife. I'm hurt, angry, and frustrated, but
> the only thing I can do is try to eat my troubles away.

Some of these men expect their wives to join them in perpetuating the myth of their sexual adequacy. "My husband is quite happy as an impotent man," one wife wrote: "He never touches me, has no idea how I feel, and isn't interested in finding out. He is charming around other women and can't keep his hands off them, so no one would guess he has a problem. They think I'm lucky to be married to such a 'tiger.' If only they knew . . ."

Husbands' lack of desire is often the principal complaint of couples seeking sex therapy. Since the partner who wants the least contact generally controls a couple's sex life, wives often feel manipulated by their disinterested husbands:

> Even at the start of our marriage, we rarely had inter-
> course more than once or twice a month. I realized quite
> early that what I had deduced as the "nice" and "respect-
> ful" side of my husband was really his hesitancy about
> engaging in sex. As early as our second year together, I

was informed that I would have to bring my strong sexual desires down to his low level.

Dissatisfaction with the quality of lovemaking is another common complaint, and women are in total agreement about what it takes to be a good sex partner. The ideal lover engages in sexual foreplay, is affectionate both in and out of bed, and realizes that sex should please *both* partners.

Foreplay is extremely important. Many wives feel their husbands are oblivious to the fact that women are different from men and need a different kind of stimulation in order to reach orgasm. In describing what she sees as her husband's selfish attitude, one woman wrote:

> I am not as satisfied sexually as I would like to be because my husband doesn't take the time and effort our lovemaking deserves. I know some of this is due to his 50-plus hour week on a high pressure job, but I feel that if he were the one who wanted more than just intercourse to achieve orgasm, we'd be putting in overtime in bed.

Apart from the physical incompleteness of sex without foreplay, women can feel emotionally discounted by the experience. One woman said that her husband's refusal to acknowledge her frequent requests for certain caresses and fondling left her feeling as though "he has a great desire for *sex* without much desire for *me*."

Some women react to their husbands' disregard for their sexual needs by becoming sexually withdrawn. Others try to be sexually accommodating in the hope that one day the favor will be returned. But as long as they feel sexually dissatisfied, they are vulnerable to more fattening sources of satisfaction.

While some wives tolerate sexual frustration without complaint, few silently endure a general lack of intimacy in their marriages. Women agree that affectionate words and gestures are more important—and less available—than sexual intercourse. In fact, disagreement about what intimacy means and how it is expressed is the greatest wedge between husbands and wives.

In his study of male intimacy,[6] Michael McGill observed that most men think intercourse itself is proof of intimacy. They believe that further expressions of tenderness are unnecessary, irrelevant, and even undesirable. But women feel differently. In McGill's words:

> Just as intimacy is not solely expressed sexually, so sexual expression is not limited to the sex act. Women are much more conscious of this than men are. Husbands who do not express their sexual selves other than through intercourse (and husbands engage in remarkably few non-intercourse-oriented physical sexual expressions) are experienced by their wives as limited lovers . . .

This is an understatement: the chances are that they are also regarded as limited husbands.

Are men incapable of being tender and romantic? Some may be. But most were attentive and tender during courtship, and wives of these men feel deceived when the caresses and sweet words of courtship all but vanish after marriage.

It's even worse when a woman believes she was the victim of deliberate courtship deception. She may believe that her husband only went through the motions of being loving, knowing full well he would drop his "act" once they were married. As the wife sees it, her husband thinks marriage entitles him to sex on demand, without his having to woo her each time they make love. Understandably, this leaves her feeling unloved and unappreciated: "I often try to give him a hug or a kiss, but he usually pushes me away. How can he care so little about my feelings? All I want is an occasional physical sign that I matter to him."

It's not always easy to convince husbands that sexual intercourse is not an isolated event in the day. When we see couples in therapy, we tell them that seduction should begin with the way they say "good morning." A woman who feels loved and cared for throughout the day is much more likely to respond to sexual overtures at night (or any other time). When tender words are whispered only during intercourse, they fall on disbelieving ears: "My husband can only be affectionate while we're having sex. When it's over, so is any sign of his caring. I long for a man who would show me that he loves me on a more constant basis."

For some men, receiving affection can be just as hard as giving it. Physical expressiveness is considered to be a prelude to sex, so if they're not interested in intercourse, they rebuff signs of affection from their wives. As one woman put it, "My husband has sex with me only when *he* wants to. And that's the only time that touching is allowed. When I reach over to touch him, he tells me he's too tired or sick or something else, even if all I want to do is cuddle and be close for a few minutes. His rejection hurts so much."

Such yearning for cuddling and tenderness has reached epidemic proportions. In her January 15, 1984 column, Ann Landers asked her readers: "Would you be content to be held close and treated tenderly and forget about 'the act'?" She received over 100,000 replies, and said that in her 30 years of writing the column, she had never met with such a staggering response to any issue. The significant results? Seventy-two percent of the women said they would prefer affection and tenderness without intercourse over sexual intercourse itself.

Of course there are many reasons why women might forgo sex for affection. Some dislike their husbands, and want as little contact as possible. Some might opt for affection over sex if they had to make a choice, but prefer to have both. And others simply don't enjoy sex. But all the variations don't negate the fact that wives all over the country are longing for more love and affection.

In response to this longing, some women seek counseling with their husbands, and learn how to make their marriages better. Others end their marriages, deciding that husbands who aren't good lovers aren't worth keeping. Still other women stay married, but turn to other men for what they've been missing.

Finally, many women stay married, faithful . . . and frustrated. These women have to find ways to cope, and many turn to overeating. Food eases the misery, by providing a "reward" that doesn't have to be earned or granted, just taken. And it redirects attention from the relationship to the refrigerator.

When food habitually fills in for love, a transformation takes place. Feelings of emotional and sexual deprivation become confused with physical hunger. That confusion has its advantages; the desire for food can be satisfied without having to rely on a husband, or anyone else.

Unfortunately, the use of food to control emotions can become addictive. Once established, the pattern is extremely hard to break. "I know I'm too fat," one woman wrote, "I want to stop eating, but right now I feel like I'm starving. I want to be held and loved so badly I hurt physically. Food is the only thing that helps numb the pain. I think if I stopped overeating I would die."

When eating is used as a long-term solution to sexual and emotional frustration, the pounds can add up at a startling rate. The average woman might feel physical hunger three or four times a day, but emotional hunger might be her constant companion. When deprivation permeates her life, constant eating is an attempt to fill the emotional void:

> My husband lost interest in any kind of physical or
> sexual intimacy with me five years ago. I learned to live

with the frustration by consoling myself with cookies, doughnuts, and other sweets. Whenever I felt like being touched, I stifled the desire with any sweets I could find. Eventually, I stopped needing physical contact, but my desire for food is now so uncontrollable that I've ballooned up to 187 pounds!

As we see, eating to cope with sexual frustration eventually causes more problems than it solves. Women don't want to be fat, they just want some relief from situations they feel powerless to control. But once they gain weight, they feel even less in control. Overeating makes them feel even more helpless and frustrated. But as long as food is the only thing that makes life bearable, there's no point in trying to give it up. The rewards of overeating are more powerful than the weight problems it creates.

HOW IS A BAD MARRIAGE
LIKE A HOT FUDGE SUNDAE?

Any marriage can be fattening, but an unhappy marriage can have an extraordinary effect. Happily married women in our survey had an average weight gain of 18.4 pounds in 13 years, while those who were in unhappy marriages gained 42.6 pounds . . . more than 2 1/2 times as much! And while 35 percent of the happily married women reached their goal weights at least once, only 2.5 percent of the women in distressed marriages could make this claim.

To avoid jumping to premature conclusions, we considered a number of plausible explanations for these differences. It was possible that unhappy wives had major weight problems before marriage. If so, they may have had fewer marital choices, and "settled for less" when choosing a mate.

Plausible, but not true. On the average, there was only a five-pound difference between the wedding day weights of happily vs. unhappily married women. Those extra five pounds weren't nearly enough to account for the eventual major weight disparity between the two groups.

Other possible explanations were also ruled out. Women who stayed home gained more weight than those who held outside jobs, but not nearly enough to account for the effects of marital unhappiness. Women with less education, lower family income, and/or more children had a little more trouble controlling their weight, but the differences were negligible compared to those associated with a bad marriage.

Careful analysis of these and other findings leads to an inescapable conclusion: *unhappy marriages are very powerful in compounding weight problems.* Marital distress can produce the kind of weight gains one would expect from a diet of hot fudge sundaes.

This conclusion holds for men as well as women. Based on wives' reports of their husbands' weight gains, husbands in the happiest marriages gained an average of 19 pounds. In sharp contrast, men in the worst marriages averaged weight gains of 38 pounds.

Great care must be taken in interpreting these statistics: *the fact that a woman is obese does not necessarily mean she's in a bad marriage.* Indeed, over 75 percent of the overweight women in our research considered their marriages to be happy. But the rest were in marriages that ranged from fairly to extremely *un*happy. More often than not, these were the women with the most recalcitrant weight problems.

We see this connection in our therapeutic work. Typically, when a woman asks us for help in losing weight, she recounts her weight history in great detail. She'll begin with her first major weight gain, continue with descriptions of failed diet and exercise attempts, and punctuate her story with expressions of self-contempt and desperation. Though she won't mention her husband until we ask, our query is often followed by a long tale of a sad marriage.

Take Gwen, for example. By the time she joined our weight loss group, she had already spent 20 fruitless years trying to get back down to her pre-marriage weight of 110 pounds. Still, she was convinced that all she needed was the "right" diet. She had tried every diet and every weight loss organization on the market. Her only success was with a clinic that insisted on daily visits during which they gave her pills and exhorted her to follow a 500 calorie diet. Gwen was able to tolerate this regimen of deprivation and obsession for five weeks. When she gave up, she was thoroughly depleted of energy, money, and any hope of reaching her goal weight.

Gwen attributed her weight problem to a late-in-life pregnancy, and a knee problem that made exercise difficult. She never mentioned marital problems, and when we asked her about her marriage, she gave us a look that said "What business is that of yours?" We explained that sometimes husbands intentionally or unintentionally play a role in their wives' weight problems, and that we'd like to understand how her husband might be helping or hindering her efforts.

Gwen sighed, and stared at the floor. Then in a voice just above a whisper, she said:

> He doesn't deliberately hurt me, but he has a habit of "fooling around" with other women. I don't know if it's been one woman for the last twenty years, or a series of different lovers. But he's away from home most of the time, and refuses to account for where he's been.
>
> Sometimes he says he's playing golf, but a few times I drove to the golf course to check for his car, and it's

never there. Other times he says he's going for a drive. But one day I set the odometer, and found that in the three hours he was gone, he drove exactly seven miles. He could have walked seven miles in that length of time!

Had Gwen talked to her husband about her suspicions, we asked?

Oh, I've hinted from time to time, but I've never accused him outright. I'm afraid of how he'd react. Basically, we don't talk to each other. He's not the kind of person who gets close. He's nice to me, gives me all the control of the money, never tells me what to do . . . but there's no closeness.

When he does talk to me, he usually nags me about my weight and calls me names like "toothpick" or "slim." Yet when I try to stay away from food by asking him to cook his own meals, he sits and sulks and refuses to eat. He's a meat and potatoes man, and wouldn't touch a salad if his life depended on it. I end up cooking for him because I feel so guilty making only things that I can eat. It's a losing battle. Once I tried to explain to him how he made it harder for me to lose weight, but that just made him angry.

I never binge eat, but I do find myself nibbling when I'm home. Food is my companionship and my comfort.

Gwen insisted that her husband would not join her in therapy, and she wouldn't allow us to try to persuade him to change his mind. We couldn't intervene without her permission, so the much-needed marriage therapy was, and is, out of the question. Meanwhile, Gwen continues to search for the magic diet. But we suspect that until she solves her marital problems, her weight will continue to torment her.

Many other women described their use of food to satisfy needs their husbands ignore. One common complaint focused on alcoholic husbands: "Once he reaches for the bottle, I know he's lost to me for the rest of the night. I've faced the fact that I won't be able to change him, but I have to do something to help me cope with my feelings of disappointment and sadness. So while he drinks, I eat." Wives of alcoholics feel acutely isolated and helpless to change their husbands. Eventually, some discover that they've become as addicted to food as their husbands have to drink.

Drinking is often compounded by occasional or frequent physical abuse. One-fifth of the women in our research reported at least one instance of domestic violence. Generally, the abuse was a one-time occurrence. But for some women, it was a regular event.

Again, eating offers some small comfort. Here is just one description of how an abused wife consoled herself with food: "I do everything I can to keep him pleased and happy, but most of the time I fail. And when I do, he gets mad, he beats me up, and then goes out all night. When he's out, I eat. When he's home, he drinks and I eat. When I get hit, I cry, and when I cry I eat. I guess eating's the best friend I have. I sure wish I had a good man instead."

A more subtle but equally destructive form of abuse is the verbal insult that attempts to keep women insecure and submissive:

> He loves to put me down in front of people and complains constantly about my cooking, housekeeping, appearance—and anything else he can think of. When other people say the meal was delicious, he says "she only cooks that way for company." If I try to contribute to the conversation, he tells me my ideas are stupid. If he

hears someone tell me I look good, he says "you better get your eyes checked!" He's made me feel I can't do anything right, which is probably why my weight has gone from 130 when we married to the 180 pounds I weigh today.

When women suffer at their husbands hands, it's natural for them to turn to others for help. Sometimes they find the support and assistance they need. But unfortunately, even professional helpers can be totally insensitive. One battered wife described having to be taken to the local hospital emergency room, where the physician jokingly asked what she had done to make her husband so mad. The physician's reprehensible behavior should have been reported to the authorities, but this battered wife remained silent, and wondered whether the doctor might be correct in assuming she was to blame.

Wives who tolerate their husbands' abuse always suffer psychological damage. To justify staying in abusive marriages, they have to rationalize the abuse, convincing themselves that it is somehow justified. The punishment becomes proof of the crime, and with each vilification, their self-esteem is lowered. Eventually, their humiliation is complete, as this poignant and perceptive comment shows: "I lost sight of who I was—I became the woman my husband told me no man could love."

Although women in these abusive relationships strongly suspect that their only chance for happiness is to switch instead of fight, many feel obligated to stay in terrible marriages for economic, religious, or other reasons. Some are afraid they could not find employment and become self-supporting. Others "stay together for the children," even if the children are suffering too. Finally, there are those who feel committed to the marriage sacrament, even though their husbands clearly are not: "I married for better or worse, and it has surely been the worst for me. I couldn't live with myself if I didn't honor my vows to stay married 'till death do us part,' even though my husband never intended to 'love, honor, and obey.' "

When women don't see any way either to improve or end their marriages, they're forced to deal with their problems in less direct ways. Overeating isn't the only option, but all too often it's the first and easiest choice.

III

The Many Uses of Fat
in Marriage

Most overweight women claim it's food they want, not fat. Typically they'll say: "If only someone would invent a magic pill that would let me eat as much as I want without gaining an ounce, I wouldn't have a care in the world."

Because we had naively accepted the notion that fat was never a *choice,* but instead an unwanted *consequence* of eating, our survey didn't examine the possible *benefits* of being overweight. Fortunately, many women took the time to enlighten us. We were amazed at the number of letters describing the usefulness of being fat and the pitfalls of being thin. But even as these women emphasize the benefits of being overweight, they lament being "trapped" in situations that force them to remain heavy. Being fat may seem like the best alternative, but it is never a satisfying one.

Once we understood the various benefits of being overweight, we realized why the topic is so seldom discussed. It touches on sensitive areas like infidelity, sexual dissatisfaction, anger, and most painful of all, the fear of being a failure as a person. These issues can be so threatening that they're not allowed into conscious awareness. And even the women who recognize these problems are reluctant to talk about them.

The safety of anonymous letters made it possible for our respondents to reveal their very personal anxieties and fears. We'll describe how the benefits of being overweight and the fears of being thin lead women to use food to protect themselves.

FOOD AND FIDELITY

The most commonly accepted reason for wanting to lose weight is also the number-one threat. According to the women in our study, increased sex appeal sounds much better than it is.

Some women who had lost weight were uncomfortable about increased male attention. Others were troubled by the temptation to yield to men's sexual advances. Still others had affairs they later regretted. Literally hundreds of women had disappointing or frightening sexual experiences they attributed to their weight loss, and many were determined to prevent these from ever happening again.

Let's look at the experience of Sheryl, who lost sixty pounds and eventually regained it all:

> Even when I weighed close to 200 pounds, my life was very satisfying. I had a good job, a lot of friends, and I was taking night courses at the community college. Everything was going so well that I decided I might as well tackle my last big challenge—losing weight. You can't imagine my pride when I reached my goal weight of 133 in just seven months.
>
> But being thin turned out to be a huge disappointment. As my weight loss became more and more obvious, the guys at work stopped treating me like a pal and started to treat me like some sexy chick. When I became

the target of off-color comments about my new sex appeal, I felt they no longer took me seriously. And two married men who I thought were my friends tried to proposition me. When I turned them down, they stopped talking to me.

I was deeply hurt by these experiences. It felt as though I didn't matter anymore—I had become just another body to be exploited. Because I looked good, my friendliness was interpreted as seductiveness, and I had to be defensive in dealing with almost any man. I expected to feel more a part of the world once I was thin, but instead I felt just the opposite.

I don't think I consciously chose to regain my lost weight. It was more a matter of being upset, and indulging in some of my favorite foods to cheer myself up. Well, the weight came back on even faster than it had come off, to the point that I'm almost back to my all-time high. I feel safer and freer in my fat body than I did when I looked my best. When people accept me, I know they like me for who I am, not how I look. And now I can do what I want, without being hassled by men.

Like so many other women, Sheryl discovered that weight loss completely changed how men responded to her, and she wasn't at all pleased with the change. While she had been looking forward to being more attractive, she hadn't considered the sexual and social implications of this change.

Experiences such as Sheryl's can be particularly unnerving for women who have never had much sexual attention. It takes practice to rebuff sexual propositions comfortably without taking them too seriously. For those who haven't mastered these skills, sexual attention from friends and strangers causes feelings that go beyond fright to the point of panic.

The easiest way for women like Sheryl to cope is to revert to old ways . . . and old weights. They know that life as a fat person isn't easy. But at least it's familiar, and it allows them to stay safely on the sidelines of the sexual arena.

The fear of being sexually attractive sometimes masks a deeper fear: that of being sexually promiscuous. We heard from women who claimed to have sexual appetites as immense as their hunger for food. One single woman described a common dilemma: "Usually, an overweight woman is limited in her choices for a romantic partner. After a large weight loss, she has new choices about sex and romance, and the popularity can be frightening. Fear of promiscuity may be a reason why some of us keep a marginal wall of fat for protection."

This fear can be present in both married and single women. But the married women often have more to lose by acting on their urges. Frightened by the temptation to have an extramarital affair, many deliberately use fat to suppress their sexual desires.

One woman, who had been an active member of four different weight loss organizations, conducted an informal survey of her fellow members. Her conclusion was that many overweight women have hearty appetites for sex. "They are very sensual ladies," she wrote. "Like me, many of them hide behind their obesity to avoid the guilt feelings that cheating would cause."

We don't know whether overweight women really do have stronger sex drives than thin women. But we've already seen that many women, fat or thin, are dissatisfied with the quality of sex and intimacy in their marriages. They may not want to leave their husbands, but neither are they hopeful about the possibility of making their marriages better. So they're left with a conflict between the temptation to seek outside satisfaction and the fear of the risks involved.

This may be why so many overweight wives believe that fat protects them from extramarital sex. Whether or not they've ever had an affair, they feel that being overweight lessens their desire to do so. A substantial number of our respondents believe that the appeal of extramarital sex increases when they lose weight. Weight gain weakens the desire to stray as well as the temptation to turn sexual fantasies into realities.

All of these women risk basing their decisions about extramarital sex on how much or how little they weigh! This woman's story illustrates the point:

> I know it sounds dumb, but I think one of the reasons I overeat is to be sure I'm not attractive to other men. When I am near my low weight, I get a lot of male attention, and I love it! I stick to my diet better than ever, and I flirt a lot. Then I feel guilty about my flirtations, and I start eating again. I usually regain even more than I lost, which leaves me more depressed than ever, and longing for the attention that made me feel so good.

Having little trust in her own ability to handle sexual attention, a woman may see weight gain as the easiest way to avoid being propositioned in the first place. She can also call on self-consciousness about weight to give her the strength to refuse propositions, and thereby keep her marriage stable.

Obviously, not all wives avoid extramarital sex. Among our respondents, almost 25 percent reported having had one or more affairs. Not surprisingly, those who were least happy with their marriages were three times more likely to have affairs. Wives of physically violent men were also more inclined to take lovers, as were women who felt their husbands were indifferent to their marriages.

But a bad marriage isn't a necessary precursor to extramarital sex. Some women who seem content with their husbands also embark on affairs once they lose weight. Generally, these women have been fat all their lives and want to take advantage of opportunities never before available. For example:

> Three years ago, I reached my goal weight of 122. Even though my husband was pleased and admired my new body, somehow it wasn't enough for me. My husband was the only man I had ever been intimate with, and once I had a body I was proud of, I wanted to be appreciated by other men. So I had a series of affairs, which luckily my husband never discovered. These other men gave me a new lease on life, after which I was able to return to being the "faithful wife."

So long as the rewards of the affair outweigh the consequences, women tend to keep their weight down. But when affairs end badly, or when they add to marital strain, women may decide against further involvements. Guilt, disappointment, or fear of discovery may be the primary motivation, but the challenge is the same: to find a way to resist sexual temptation. The solution is one they already know. To say "no" to other men, women say "yes" to food.

Here's just a small sampling of the various explanations women give:

> I am now 90 pounds overweight because I no longer want the secret company of my lover of nearly six years. I can't say no to him—God knows I've tried. So my subconscious method seems to be to get grossly obese so he'll lose interest.

> After my husband found out about my affair, he beat me up. Because he won't forgive and forget, I got fat again. That way he knows my lover won't want me

anymore, and, to tell the truth, I couldn't let him see me even if he did.

I lost 40 pounds two years ago, after which my husband and I started switching partners with our dearest neighbors. It destroyed our friendship with them, and it almost did our marriage in. After that, I regained all the weight I lost. I know I'm not happy carrying all this fat around. But God I'm scared to death to be without it!

These women are convinced they can't resist other men without an inhibiting layer of extra weight. Fat is a necessary prop in the role of dutiful, faithful wife.

One important question remains unanswered: Do these women consciously decide to regain weight, or do they gain the weight first, and come up with the explanation later? Since most of our letters came from women who were well above their "affair weights," we can't be sure. Based on their descriptions, it appears that some deliberately regain their weight, while others resume old habits without intending to get fat.

Those who intentionally regain their weight may be a step ahead of those who take no responsibility for their weight gain. At least they acknowledge the problem. Unfortunately, once they do regain weight, they're stuck in the same old rut, but this time it's even worse. Being thin has lost its appeal, but being fat is no fun either. The best they can expect is to find a way to blunt the pain of being fat, while avoiding the risks of being thin.

Some women who appear to gain weight "against their will" are reacting to problems raised by the affairs themselves. Because affairs are usually kept secret, women seldom turn to other people for help. And when no safe confidant is available, it's easy to turn to the one "friend" who can keep a secret . . . food.

So instead of confronting their problems, these women muffle their anxiety. When eating finally takes its toll, they may convince themselves that they "subconsciously" regained weight to avoid future affairs and the danger of being hurt. But in accepting a subconscious explanation for their behavior, they lose the chance to direct their own destiny.

Most of these women are convinced that the connection between thinness and infidelity is unavoidable. They may even believe that weight loss is the *cause* of infidelity. When they feel good about their bodies, they assume they can't help but "give in" to any man who shows interest. So they channel their desires into overeating, until they gain enough weight to feel protected from the sexual experiences they fear.

KEEPING HUSBANDS
AT A DISTANCE

Being heavy and feeling unattractive can be as useful for keeping husbands at bay as for avoiding outside attention. Many women, consciously or not, put on weight to escape marital sex. Weight gain usually serves a double purpose: it diminishes a husband's sexual interest, and it inhibits a woman's own sexual desire.

Three situations seemed to be commonly associated with an aversion to marital sex. One came as quite a shock: many wives were repelled by their husbands' fat! Because so many women in our study felt rejection due to their weight, we hardly expected them to reject their husbands for the same reason. But one-fourth of our respondents reported a decline in sexual interest when their husbands' weight went up. Almost half said their husbands' weight was the *only* cause of their own lack of sexual interest.

We were even more startled to discover what small amounts

of weight could make a difference. One woman wrote: "I don't like a 'belly' on a man, however slim he is. That's where my husband's extra 10–15 pounds settle. He's very attractive to me without the paunch, but he has no sex appeal for me when he has it."

With further thought, this phenomenon became less baffling. We realized that the average woman in our study has an aversion to fat—on herself or anyone else. Even though she feels rejected when her husband withdraws from her, she usually believes this rejection is justified. Recognizing her own weight as a sexual turnoff, it makes sense that her husband's fat is equally unappealing.

But few women feel they can speak to their husbands directly about the problem. Some have been so hurt by criticism of their weight that they can't bring themselves to judge anyone else. Others want to avoid possible conflict over such a sensitive issue. Whatever the reason, many wives decide that the easiest way to avoid marital sex is to gain or regain weight.

A second group of women lost interest in sex when it became too routine. These women, too, were reluctant to ask for changes. Some decided it was easier to give up sex altogether than try to spice up a dull sex life:

> When we first married, sex was SO thrilling and exciting—like going on a trip to the moon! Then we got accustomed to each other. The thrill has long since checked out of the bedroom, and boredom has taken its place. Going through the acrobatics of trying to make it fun is ridiculous, because if you don't enjoy sex missionary style, you won't enjoy it standing on your head. I lived the first 19 years of my life without sex, so who needs it now?

Others are so bored with their sexual routines that they prefer tasty treats to making love:

> Before we married, there was lots of hugging and kissing and fondling before intercourse. I loved the romance even more than the sex. But after marriage, he settled into a systematic routine—like a pilot checking out his aircraft: i.e. two kisses, three squeezes, a touch on each breast, two tummy rubs and ready to go! Lately, I find late night snacks much more enjoyable than sex. And if an extra ten pounds makes him less interested, so much the better.

Finally, a third group of women attempt to stifle their own desire for sex when their husbands can't or won't have intercourse. Many apparently believe it "hurts less" if they deliberately contribute to their own rejection by gaining weight. It's as if they're saying, "You can't fire me, I quit!"

These wives generally are determined to remain faithful. Initially, they overeat in an attempt to allay sexual frustration. But once they gain weight, they discover an unexpected benefit of being heavy—their own sexual interest diminishes:

> My husband stopped wanting sex after I had our second child. At first, that was fine with me, because I had gained so much weight that I didn't want him to get too close. But after I lost the weight, I started wanting sex again. Unfortunately, his desire never returned. While I was thin, I couldn't stop thinking about sex, and I stuffed myself with junk food every time he rejected me. Eventually, I got back to my high weight, and discovered, much to my relief, that my "urgent" need for sex had

disappeared. I don't like being fat, but it does make it much easier to cope with his indifference.

There is a sad assumption here that sexual problems have no solution. One might wonder why so many wives choose to deal with these problems in such an indirect way, especially since it's usually easier to improve an unsatisfying sex life than to endure it.

As we all know, however, many people are inhibited about discussing sex. Chances are that one or both partners were reared in homes where parents were too embarrassed to bring up the topic. And those couples who aren't comfortable with general discussions certainly won't admit to their own sexual concerns. Avoiding the issue altogether seems the safest (and perhaps only) solution.

A wife may also use weight gain as a form of birth control, minimizing sexual contact and the chance of becoming pregnant. We heard from one woman who attributed an unplanned pregnancy to her loss of 15 pounds. She vowed not to let it happen again: "I know I shouldn't blame the pregnancy on my weight loss, but neither my husband nor I would have had that kind of sexual desire if I had been heavier. In the future, I'll stay fat, because I don't want and we can't afford a fourth child." Given the widespread lack of knowledge about contraception, as well as certain religious prohibitions against its use, this method may not be such an unusual form of natural family planning.

Weight gain to avoid sex seems to be least common among women with the most unhappy marriages. Once wives are deeply dissatisfied, they feel less compelled to rely upon covert ways to avoid sex. They're less concerned about protecting their husbands' feelings, and they seldom have trouble just saying "No!" And since husbands in unhappy marriages are also generally less interested, the need to refuse may seldom arise.

The mildly discontented wives are the ones most likely to use their weight to create distance from husbands. To keep their marriages stable, they sacrifice not only their bodies and their sensuality, but also their self-esteem.

SWALLOWING THE ANGER

Like sex, anger is more often avoided than discussed. Most children rarely have the opportunity to watch their parents argue constructively, and girls are doubly handicapped. They're told that fighting isn't "ladylike," and are discouraged from ever learning how.

As adults, women are often accused of being unreasonable, overemotional, and even hysterical whenever they express anger. And those who are married to abusive men learn that displays of anger can lead to physical harm. Under these conditions, it's reasonable to conclude that the best way to handle anger is to "swallow" it, keeping it to oneself.

Internalized anger is often washed down with food, to make the "meal" more palatable. Although pounds accumulate as the anger builds, being overweight can make it easier to cope. One formerly fat woman described how her weight kept her passive:

> I tolerated a lot when I was fat—much more than I do now that I am thin. Because of my weight, I felt somehow undeserving of the pleasures other people enjoyed—things like a good job, nice clothes, and most importantly, a good marriage. I always tried to make myself content with less, and I never confronted my resentment, except to mask it by stuffing myself with food.

This is a major "benefit" of being fat. If a woman feels she doesn't deserve to be happy, she doesn't have to worry about finding ways to improve her life. She can even talk herself out of her anger toward others by convincing herself that she has no right to be mad at anyone but herself.

Other women gain weight to rebel against someone who wants them to be thin. Weight loss becomes a concession they're unwilling to make. One woman said, "In the years we've been married, he has done nothing to help me feel good. Why should I struggle to keep weight off because he thinks I should?" Weight gain is her way of assuring that her husband is as unhappy as she is.

A cogent illustration was provided by a client of ours, who at 5′ 6″ weighed 250 pounds. This is how she explained how she gained well over 100 pounds since her marriage:

> I never had a weight problem as a girl, although I thought I did. I was 112 pounds when I got my drivers license, and I lied about my weight because I thought I was too fat.
>
> I was still 112 when I met my husband. From the day we were engaged, he was after me about what I ate. He was terrified about having a fat wife—his mother was quite fat—and he watched me like a hawk whenever I ate anything. It made me so mad . . . and it still does. I wanted to say to him: "I'm an adult; I've handled my weight all these years without your help—what makes you think suddenly I need to be told what to eat?"
>
> So I finally figured "If I can't eat while he's here, I'll eat when he's not around." I didn't want to fight with him, so it was easier just to go behind his back. I did a lot of sneak-eating during my gaining years. I could hide what I ate in closets and boxes, but of course it eventually showed up on my body.

During the twenty years of our marriage, he's been like a policeman—giving me lectures if I go off a diet for a day. I'm surprised he doesn't fine me! Anyway, the more he nags, the madder I get. If I *do* watch what I eat, I feel as though I'll be giving in to him. My only way of fighting back is to stay fat. But neither of us is happy with this solution.

When a woman's weight is a major issue in her marriage, her body becomes the battleground in a power struggle no one wins. By staying fat, she has the satisfaction of knowing she's not "giving in" to her husband's control. But she works against her own best interests by mistakenly assuming she has to choose between being fat and independent or being subservient and thin.

FEAR OF FAILURE

A fear that's discussed far less than it's experienced is the fear of failure. It's so threatening that even in anonymous letters it's mentioned obliquely, if at all. Signs of it show up in phrases like "If only I were thin, I would . . ." or "When I lose weight, I will . . ." These expressions, when used by women who have been overweight for years, hide their fear that they won't measure up in some important area of life.

One of the most common fears is expressed by middle-aged, married women who haven't worked outside the home for many years. In the typical case, a woman whose children are grown doubts her ability to handle the "empty-nest syndrome." Fearing the challenges of the outside world, weight becomes an excuse for not taking risks. The woman won't leave the safety of her home until she's lost a sufficient amount of weight . . . but she never loses enough to take that first step.

Lillian's story illustrates this dilemma:

> I've been fat for so long that I've forgotten what it's like to be any other way. It seems I've spent my whole life in this house—looking after the kids, cleaning, cooking, and baking. And eating . . . lots of eating.
>
> Sometimes I fantasize about what life would be like if I lost 50 pounds. I wouldn't be ashamed to be seen in public, so I'd go out more. I'd get some kind of job— God knows we could use the money. But I've never been anything but a housewife, so I doubt anybody would hire me. And I've suffered so much disapproval because of my fat, it would kill me to be rejected by employers too. I can't face going out and competing with all those thin, confident women. I know I'd lose.

Lillian's fears may be realistic. It *is* difficult to enter the job market with few or no marketable skills. And prejudice against obesity is not a figment of her imagination; weight loss probably would make it easier for her to get a job.

But Lillian was also afraid of challenge and change. Losing weight would rob her of her major excuse for clinging to the security of her home. It would force her to confront her fears and try to overcome them, and Lillian just wasn't ready to take that step.

These fears can escalate and become the dominant focus of women's lives. When signs of true agoraphobia result, women will need professional help, not weight loss, before they can overcome the anxiety that keeps them "safe" inside the home.

A weight problem can also mask fears of marital failure; it

justifies a husband's disinterest, and even abuse. A woman can postpone or avoid trying to improve her marriage by fixating on weight. She guarantees that she will remain insecure: telling herself that her weight would keep her from finding another man or becoming financially and emotionally independent, she tolerates a level of unhappiness she'd never put up with if she felt better about herself.

Jeanine, a member of one of our weight loss groups, realized that she was using her fat to avoid leaving her alcoholic husband. Because she was addicted to food, she rationalized that she had no right to complain about his addiction to alcohol. And because her weight magnified her feelings of insecurity, she couldn't imagine striking out on her own. Her weight problem allowed her to distract herself from her husband's problem, over which she had no control, and focus her attention on her own failings. This obviously didn't make her happy, but it did allow her to avoid the challenge of reestablishing herself as a single woman.

Weight often becomes a convenient scapegoat for other problems in a woman's life. She can look to calories instead of counseling as the cure for her ills. And she can console herself by saying *"fat is the problem, it isn't me!"* For beneath most fears of failure in marriage or work lies a more basic fear: that of not being worthwhile as a person.

Insecurity is most common among women who were fat as teenagers, just when they were most eager to conform and most vulnerable to rejection for being different. Because they usually felt responsible for their excess weight, the rejection seemed deserved.

Years of conditioning can lead a woman to connect overweight with failure, and the linkage between weight and self-esteem creates a self-fulfilling prophesy. Here's the typical pattern:

- Because she's fat, she doesn't compete;
- Because she doesn't compete, she can't win;
- With no successes to her credit, she feels bad about herself;
- The worse she feels, the more she eats, and the heavier she grows;
- And with each pound she gains, her self-esteem falls even further.

Once caught in this cycle, a woman can become blind to everything except her weight problem. Instead of taking action no matter what her weight, she pins her hopes on losing weight as the *only* way to set everything right.

Why, then, doesn't she lose weight? Well, she's not at all sure she can succeed. Losing weight would put her to the test—a test she'll probably fail. And failure would only further weaken her self-esteem. It's easier to stay fat and dream of being thin; that at least leaves room for fantasies of success.

As if this isn't bad enough, even weight loss *success* can hold a threat of personal failure. Women in our weight loss groups have expressed fears of what might be expected of them if they do lose weight. One of the group members shared this apprehension:

> When I'm fat, people expect so little of me that there's no way I can disappoint them. In fact, expecting so little, they're often impressed by what I actually can do.
> I don't know if people would be as impressed if I were thin. I wonder if I could live up to their beliefs about what a thin woman should be. It would be devastating to discover I'm only impressive "for a fat lady."

Clearly, weight can shelter women from a wide range of fears. It allows them to withdraw from difficult and painful challenges by restricting their attention to the circumscribed areas of food and body size. What most of these women are saying is: "I can't lose if I don't play the game." By staying on the fringes of life, they avoid the pain of losing. But they also give up any chance of winning.

IV

Husbands Who Fatten
Their Wives

We've heard countless stories of husbands who create and perpetuate their wives' weight problems. The variety of techniques would make good copy for a self-help manual for husbands intent on keeping their wives "Fat for Life."

When we first heard these stories, we wondered if the husbands were being unfairly blamed. But when we invited the men to join their wives for counseling, we found that many were guilty as charged. And the strategies they used were both ingenious and relentless.

Whenever interference is deliberate, it's important to understand not only *how* a husband stymies his wife's weight loss, but also *why* he feels it necessary to do so. We'll examine the most common tactics, as well as the motives behind them.

HOW TO PREVENT
A WIFE'S WEIGHT LOSS

One of the most effective ways to prevent a wife from losing weight is to demand that she do so. At least that seems to be the consensus of the women who wrote to us. Nothing is more irritating to a wife than a husband who tries to pressure her into losing weight. She's likely to see his insistence as coercive, insulting, and rejecting. And in fact, it often is.

Take, for example, this story of a woman who felt victimized by her husband's unending demands:

> A month after our marriage, my husband suggested we both go on diets. That was the start of 26 years of nagging about my weight, which is never low enough to suit him. When I weighed 135, he thought I should lose 10 pounds. When I weighed 123, he thought 115 would be better. After I used all the tricks of anorexics to reach 115, he said I still looked too fat.
>
> That was when I snapped! I couldn't take it anymore, because I finally realized I could never please him. So now I'm up to 166. Since he's going to think I'm fat no matter what I weigh, I might as well relax and eat whatever I want.

Stories like this are not uncommon. Many wives initially try to meet their husbands' demands for weight loss, no matter how unrealistic the demands might be. Since most women in our thin-obsessed culture feel fat no matter how much they weigh, criticism from a loved one only confirms their belief that they must lose weight to be acceptable. As one wife said: "When the person who's supposed to love me the most thinks I'm too fat to be lovable, I figure I must be really bad."

Only when the hoped-for acceptance fails to materialize even after major weight losses, do women start to suspect that their weight may not be the real issue. At that point, some women regain weight, while others decide to look for new men.

A less direct, but equally cruel, form of pressure involves

comparisons with other women. Instead of dealing with the issue straightforwardly, some husbands throw out hurtful hints. In the words of a wife on the receiving end:

> It doesn't bother me too much when my husband calls me out of the kitchen to admire a lovely actress on television. But when he refers to a Miss America type as "that fat chick," I naturally get upset. I weigh 130 pounds and I'm less than 5 feet tall. I can't get much thinner, and I'll certainly never be tall. If the thinks these women are fat and dumpy, what can he think of me?

Another woman described how inadequate she felt when her husband made remarks about various women waiting in line with them at the movie theater. A typical comment was: "If you had legs like hers, I might still be attracted to you." Needless to say, this scarcely put the wife in the frame of mind to lose weight.

We also heard from women whose husbands had affairs . . . and then let their wives know that the "other women" were thin. Some of these wives were infuriated, but others blamed themselves for being so fat that their husbands were "forced" to stray.

Another common tactic of husbands is constant criticism. Too many spouses are under the illusion that nagging and criticism will eventually cause mates to change. Actually, nagging only intensifies problems:

> My husband is always bugging me to lose weight, but he's never satisfied with my efforts. When I take the exact portion size my diet requires, he tells me I'm eating too much. When I eat legal snacks, he tells me I'm being a pig. And as I slowly sip my glass of ice water, while I watch him devour a bag of potato chips and guzzle down

a six-pack, I have to listen to his lectures about exercise.
His constant put-downs only make it harder for me to
stick to my diet.

A husband who nags and criticizes will all but guarantee that
his wife will nourish her weight problem. Some men don't
realize this, and get increasingly frustrated—and critical—when
their efforts seem in vain. But as we'll see, other men are fully
aware of what they are doing. They want their wives to fail,
and they use that failure to justify and intensify their own harsh
criticism.

Another weapon in the husbands' arsenal is the mixed message,
which is the confusing communication of two incompatible
desires. Typically, a husband will say he wants his wife to lose
weight, but act in a way that tells her to stay heavy. For example,
a husband may insist that his wife lose weight, but complain
when she tries to serve the family low-calorie meals. Or he may
suggest that she start to exercise, and then gripe about expenses
when she wants to join a health club or buy an exercise bike.

We saw an interesting use of mixed messages by the husband
of a woman we were treating for life-threatening obesity. This
couple seemed to have a very good marriage, and the husband
appeared to be supportive of his wife's weight-loss efforts. But
when it became clear that she would never lose weight as long
as she was home full-time, the husband changed his tune. "A
mother should be home to greet her children when they return
from school," he exclaimed. When the wife went ahead and took
a full-time job (and started to lose weight), he became increasingly critical. He worried that the children were being neglected,
and her job was "too stressful." In response to his barrage, the
wife started to feel guilty. Eventually, she quit her job and
returned to her daily routine of baking chocolate chip cookies

"for the children." She ate most of the cookies before her children walked through the front door.

Mixed messages create a no-win situation. Because contradictory requests have been made, any response is the wrong one. Whether women gain or lose weight, they can be punished for their choice. Unable to figure out what their husbands really want, many women decide the easiest choice is to stay fat.

A husband's sabotage can take many forms. He can:

· Demand that his wife prepare fattening meals she can't resist;
· Insist on keeping "forbidden" treats within easy reach;
· Urge her to share high-calorie snacks that are not part of her diet;
· Offer to do the grocery shopping, and then buy all the wrong foods;
· Bring home gifts of sweets as a reward for weight loss;
· Complain about being lonely when she leaves the house to exercise;
· Complain about the expense of exercise equipment, health club memberships, aerobics classes, etc.

These are the common sabotage techniques, but they are far from the most creative, or the most destructive. The truly insidious tactics involve switching the focus from food to other matters that are less obviously connected to weight loss. This makes it harder for a wife to pinpoint or confront the sabotaging behavior. Here's an illustration:

> My husband claims he doesn't care what I weigh, but every time I lose weight, he lays into me . . . not about weight . . . but about everything else under the sun. He

complains about my housekeeping, my friends, and my general attitude. He makes my life so miserable that I turn to food for comfort. As I start to gain weight, he relaxes.

I've tried to point this out to him, but he tells me I'm crazy. He says he never complains about the money I spend for my weight loss program, and he's never tempted me to break my diet. I have to admit that's true, which leaves me wondering if it's all in my imagination. And yet, this has happened many times before, and the pattern is undeniable.

A husband's sabotaging behavior sometimes includes violence, as this terrifying account illustrates:

My husband wants me to look like Twiggy. For ten years, he has been threatening to lock the refrigerator or tie me up until I lose forty pounds. But the one time I almost reached my goal, he was even meaner than usual. He squeezed and pinched me, threw things at me, and even punched me one night.

When I'm fat he abuses me emotionally, but the abuse gets physical when I'm thin. I've decided it hurts less to be fat.

Unfortunately, this kind of situation is far from unique. Of the women in our study who had suffered physical abuse, most said abuse was more frequent when they were *losing* weight than when they were *gaining*. For these women, avoiding physical harm is certainly a powerful incentive to stay overweight, no matter how much their husbands insist they would like them to be thin.

Almost any attempt to coerce wives to lose weight is bound

to fail. Still, husbands persist in their efforts. This leads many women to suspect—often quite accurately—that their husbands have compelling reasons to keep them fat.

THE BENEFITS
OF HAVING A FAT WIFE

It's hard to find a man who will admit to wanting a fat wife. When directly confronted with his sabotaging actions, he's likely to declare: "I would never do anything to interfere with her weight loss . . . why should I?"

There may not be any good reasons why he *should,* but we found five good reasons why he *does.* Based not only on wives' reports, but also on our clinical observation, these are the major factors that can motivate a man to keep his wife fat:

1. Unwillingness to change comfortable daily routines;
2. Unwillingness to tackle his own weight problem;
3. Unwillingness to overcome his other bad habits such as drinking or gambling;
4. Use of weight to divert attention from marital and sexual problems;
5. Fear of a wife's infidelity.

The most common complaint focuses on husbands' unwillingness to change their own daily routines to adjust to their wives' weight-loss programs. These husbands may sincerely want their wives to lose weight, but they don't see any reason why their own lives should be affected.

These men are often accustomed to snack foods and rich desserts, and they're unwilling to forgo these pleasures "just" to help their wives. Some expect to be waited on by their wives, and won't even prepare their own snacks, much less their meals. Others don't want to give up high-calorie restaurant meals. All of these men expect their wives to continue the familiar routine, while somehow also managing to lose weight. "My husband is thrilled that I'm finally trying to diet," one woman wrote:

> The problem is that he doesn't want me to change anything but my weight. That means I'm expected to continue to buy junk food for him, and all his poker-playing friends. He also expects me to keep up our tradition of Friday night pizza, even though pizza isn't on my diet. When I tell him we have to change some of our habits, he tells me that *he* doesn't have a weight problem and that I should learn to use more self-control.

Resistance to new eating patterns is even greater when the husband also has a weight problem, especially if he has little interest in losing weight. He may sabotage his wife's weight loss in order to maintain a comfortable weight balance in the marriage.

This was the dilemma facing Chris, a client of ours with a severe weight problem. When her doctor told her she had to lose weight, Chris vowed to adhere to a strict diet and exercise regimen. She never thought that her husband would interfere with her efforts:

> My husband was very supportive at first. Since he also needed to lose, he said he'd join me in the program and we'd lose weight together. But after a week of salads and diet soda, he'd had it with dieting. He told me I was on my own. He also told me I'd have to start cooking separate meals each night. I went along because he's the breadwinner, even though it was hard to resist picking at the foods I wasn't supposed to eat.

Well, I managed to lose some weight, though not as quickly as I would have liked. And then my husband started doing weird things. One evening, he brought home a bag of treats. Another time, he baked a batch of cookies, something he had never done in his life! After that it was a series of pies, ice-cream bars, everything he could think of to get me to go off my diet. After a while, I gave up. I just couldn't fight it anymore.

An overweight husband is likely to become more and more uneasy as his wife loses weight. The implication is that if she can do it, so can he. If he stays fat, she may feel superior, which could upset the power balance in the marriage. She may also find him less acceptable sexually, which would only magnify his feelings of insecurity.

A wife's weight can establish a balance for thin husbands too. In what amounts to a tradeoff of vices, a husband may encourage his wife to overeat so he can justify continuing his own bad habits. Alcoholism is a prime example, as this woman illustrates:

My husband has his first drink with breakfast, and his last one as he drifts off each night. I have my first cinnamon roll at breakfast, and fall asleep with cookie crumbs in the bed.

Every time my husband sees me throw out all the sweets, he gets nervous. He tells me I don't need to lose any weight, and he tries to tempt me to overeat. I think he's really worried that I'll start to criticize him about his drinking. He's afraid that if I conquer my problem, I'll expect him to conquer his.

A strong dependency on nicotine can present similar problems. One husband agreed that if his wife lost weight, he'd quit smoking. But as she started to shed her extra pounds, he was unwilling —or unable—to give up cigarettes. In order to avoid keeping his part of the deal, he pressured his wife to give up her diet.

Weight problems also distract attention from marital and sexual problems. As we've seen earlier, a husband may attribute his lack of interest or performance to his wife's excess weight. This ploy is usually effective . . . that is until she starts to lose weight. She may discover that her thinner body still fails to arouse her husband's interest. Only then does she realize that weight may have simply been a cover-up for other problems.

One of the more extreme examples of this came from a woman who told of her husband's long-term impotence, which he ascribed entirely to her weight problem:

> For years he refused to have sex with me, claiming that he only found slender women attractive. Believing this, I worked hard at losing weight, and actually got to three pounds *under* goal. But he still says I'm too fat. Currently he points to his secretary who is 5′ 10″ and weighs 115 pounds as a woman that he finds sexy.

Fortunately, rather than starving herself, this woman finally figured out that her husband's impotence, not her weight, was the central issue.

Some of the saddest letters we received described husbands who used their wives' weight for a dual purpose: not only did they withdraw sexually, but they also took lovers. They regarded their behavior as a perfectly legitimate reaction to wives they considered too fat. From the wife's point of view:

> I've been trying to get rid of about 30 pounds for five years now, because my husband says my weight has caused him to lose all sexual interest in me. But every

time I start to lose, he gets even more distant, if that's possible. Instead of cheering me on, he makes snide remarks and says I'll never be able to stick to my diet.

Last month, I finally discovered what was behind all this. A neighbor told me my husband had been involved with another woman for almost seven years! At first I didn't believe it, but a little investigation proved it to be true (though he will deny it to his death . . . which couldn't come soon enough for me).

Now I understand why he wants me to be fat and ugly and insecure. He wants an excuse to stay with this other "lady," and still keep me home doing his cooking, cleaning, and laundry. But I've decided enough is enough. I'm more determined than ever to reach my goal.

Whether or not a husband is having an affair, he may discover that his wife demands much less of him when she is insecure about being overweight. If he has little interest in working to maintain a good relationship, keeping his wife fat may keep her off his back. Chances are, she'll even rationalize that she deserves the neglect.

The final motive for sabotaging weight loss is a husband's fear of his wife's infidelity. This fear is quite common, and it drives men to use tactics that are as extreme as they are effective.

A wife's awareness of this fear is often acquired painfully. One such experience was described by Linda, one of our group members. Linda is an attractive, outgoing woman who is four dress sizes larger than she'd like to be. She's not comfortable with her extra weight, but has abandoned any attempt to lose it. Her story explains why:

Last year, I made a New Year's resolution to lose the 17 pounds I'd accumulated during the first eight years of marriage. I started swimming every day, and I gave up sweets and other snack food. It took a while for the weight to come off, but by summer, I looked really great, if I do say so myself.

But just as I was feeling good, my marriage started coming apart. At first, my husband just made little "teasing" comments like: "You look so good that I don't want to let you out of my sight." I thought it was his way of complimenting me, but now I see he was feeling insecure.

His comments turned nasty by mid-summer. He hinted that I was running around behind his back, and I had to account for every minute I was away from him. He also started bringing home ice cream and candy, and telling me that I had to quit dieting and start eating like a normal person again. When I refused, he accused me of wanting to be thin "for someone else."

I told him he was crazy, and that I had lost weight for me. And I managed to resist the tempting treats and ignore his insults.

That's when he started coming home later and later, and snapping at me when I asked where he'd been. Soon I was convinced that *he* was being unfaithful, and I got very upset. Eventually I became so depressed that I lost all my willpower and went back to overeating. Soon I moved my old "fat" clothes from the basement back to my closet.

As my fat returned, so did my husband. He's his old self again, and he acts like nothing ever happened. I'm relieved, but I'm also angry at him. I understand that he was insecure—though he had no reason to be—and that he was probably afraid of losing me. But if he really loves me so much, why can't he find a better way to express his insecurity?

"Insecure" is the word used most often to describe the husband who wants his wife to be overweight. Linda's story is just one example of how a wife's increased attractiveness and self-confidence can trigger a husband's panic. His jealous comments were a sign that he feared losing this "new" woman to another man. Instead of talking about his feelings, and asking for reassurance, he began to coerce her to return to a higher, and in his mind, safer weight.

Women in these situations often choose weight gain as the most effective way to end the conflict. But they aren't happy about being fat again . . . it's merely the lesser of two evils.

Of course, sometimes a husband's fear of infidelity is realistic. As we've explained, many women feel that past affairs could be attributed to their weight loss. Being thin and more confident motivated them to find more appreciative lovers. As one woman said: "It makes me sick when I think of all those years that I was having an affair with food instead of with a real man."

Some women only turn to other men if their husbands fail to cooperate in improving the marriage. But others have so many grievances that they aren't willing to give their husbands another chance. As one woman wrote:

> I experienced many rebuffs, rejections, and exploitations as a fat woman. When I lost weight, I was emotionally available for an intimate experience—one I didn't even try to find with my husband, because he was one of the people who made me feel bad in my fat life.

The phrase "in my fat life" is significant. The physical, emotional, and social changes that accompany weight loss can be so dramatic that a woman's entire life can change. The insecure, passive, fat person of the past often bears no relationship to the confident, active, thin person of the present. And the man that the fat woman chose to marry may bear no resemblance to the man the thin woman desires.

This situation was poignantly illustrated by a couple who came to us for help. Nancy admitted to having had several affairs, and now wanted a divorce. John wanted to save the marriage. Since they had never tried marriage therapy, we asked that they let us help them give the marriage one more try. Nancy was adamant in her refusal. She wanted nothing to do with her husband; in fact, she said she could hardly stand the sight of him. She explained her feelings by relating the following story:

> I was almost 100 pounds overweight while I was dating John. When he asked me to marry him, I was thrilled. I couldn't believe that a man wanted to marry me despite the way I looked. Although I don't think I was ever really in love with him, I believed it was my only chance of getting married, so I grabbed it.
>
> For eight years, I was pretty content with our relationship. We didn't talk much, and we seldom made love, but that was just fine with me. Most of the time I was so depressed about my weight that I wouldn't have been a very good conversationalist, and I was far too embarrassed about the way I looked to be interested in sex.
>
> But now I've lost 96 pounds, and everything has changed. I'm nothing like that fat woman who married John, and I want more than he is capable of offering me. I have nothing against him . . . he's a nice guy, and I'm sure he could make some woman very happy. But not me. Quite frankly, I now know I can do better, and I can't let the opportunity pass me by.

When Nancy talked about her former fat self, she seemed to be describing a stranger. It was clear to us that she wanted nothing to do with anyone or anything from her old life. As she summed it up: "When I think about how I looked, how I felt, and what I put up with, it seems like a bad dream. It felt like being in prison. Now I want to be totally free."

Would her husband have been better off working to prevent her weight loss? John said the thought never occurred to him until after he found out about her infidelity. And by that time, he had so little influence on her that any attempt would have been futile: "If she hadn't lost all that weight, she wouldn't be leaving me. If I had seen what was coming, I might have tried to convince her to stay the way she was. But there's nothing I can do about it now."

John was unable to convince his wife to regain her weight, but many other men are very successful. We were stunned by the number of women who told us they allowed themselves to be coerced by their husbands' outrageous efforts to induce weight gain. This woman, for example, responded to her husband's bizarre displays of jealousy by doing exactly what he wanted—becoming fat again:

> After I lost 60 pounds, my husband became obsessively jealous. He took away my car keys and spending money, and accompanied me everywhere—to the laundromat, grocery store, and even to my friends' homes. He also called the house when he was at work to make sure I was there, and he asked neighbors to drop in to assure that I wasn't entertaining men during the day.

This woman truly believed that she could only maintain her weight loss with her husband's support. When his jealousy became too much for her, she decided the cost of being thin was too high.

When other tactics don't work, a jealous husband may resort

to physical abuse in an attempt to make his wife gain weight. Some wives comply, regaining their weight to stop the abuse. But others refuse to sacrifice their attractiveness and self-confidence just to pacify an insecure husband:

> My husband's physical abuse began after more than 10 years of marriage, just a few months after I lost the last of my 80 extra pounds. Once I lost weight, other men complimented me on my appearance, I got a job and financial independence, and I began to think of myself as a person in my own right instead of just as his wife and our children's mother. These things made him worry that I would leave him for another man, so he started making accusations and pushing me around. I know if I put back those 80 pounds, his abuse would stop. But I'll give up my marriage before I'll go back to being fat!

The choice doesn't always have to be either gaining weight or leaving the marriage. There are women who manage to maintain their weight losses while they work with their husbands to improve their marriage. Sad to say, we received only a few examples of this kind of resolution. Here is one:

> After I lost over 40 pounds and felt very much like a different person, my husband became so jealous that he moved out of our bedroom into the guest room. I, in turn, acted like a spoiled child and stayed away from him as much as possible. Whenever I'd come home, there he would be, munching away on all the foods that are "red light items" for me. He'd ignore me completely, and tell the kids how selfish their mother was being.
> After weeks of this, I decided we shouldn't let a good marriage pass this way, so we started talking. Within two

months, we have fallen back in love with each other. My
husband now enjoys a thinner, prettier, more self-assured
me, and he is even pleased (although I feel awkward)
when other men's heads turn.

Although this approach has the advantage of saving both the
woman's self-esteem and her marriage, it seems to be the excep-
tion. This may be due to the common, but often erroneous, belief
among spouses that the partner is unwilling or unable to change.
Because of this misperception, most wives confronted by "fattening husbands" decide they have to choose between regaining their
weight or leaving their marriages.

A note of caution is in order here. There's no question that
husbands often actively interfere with their wives' weight-loss
attempts. But it's important to realize that not every husband
who sabotages his wife's weight loss does so intentionally: husbands often act more out of ignorance than malice. They may not
know how to help, or they may be unaware of how much
influence they can have. In the final chapter, we'll offer suggestions for showing these husbands how to do it right.

V

Giving Up
the Victim Role

A paradox confronts us every time a woman seeks our help for a weight problem. She invariably begins by telling us how desperately she wants to lose weight. But before we can express our willingness to help, she explains why she's doomed to be forever fat.

Take Debby, for example. A chronic dieter, she had been overweight since her early teens. At the first session of our weight loss group, Debby launched into her story.

A fat child of fat parents, Debby felt the cards had been stacked against her from the beginning. Her mother was an immigrant who spoke little English, and who spent most of her time at home, cooking and baking. Debby thought her mother may have intentionally kept her fat and insecure so she would stay at home and keep her mother company. Whether or not the plan was deliberate, it worked.

After Debby finished high school, she found a job, left home, and with constant vigilance, managed to lose almost 40 pounds. For the first time in her life, men paid attention to her. Initially she was flattered and excited, but she didn't know how to handle the sexual demands. The internal conflict was so stressful that she began to overeat. The weight returned rapidly, and soon the men were looking elsewhere.

When she was in her mid-20s, Debby met a man who looked beyond her weight and asked her to marry him. Debby didn't love this man, but she felt it was her only chance to have children, so she said "yes." The marriage was not a happy one, and Debby gained an additional 30 pounds due to the stress of being a dissatisfied wife and an overtaxed mother.

When Debby finished her story, she shrugged her shoulders and said: "I hate being fat, but it seems like I'm doomed to stay this way."

We've heard stories like this thousands of times. A woman's case for why weight loss is impossible usually includes: a history of past failures; a stressful environment in which overeating is her only source of relief; a body that naturally resists a lower weight; and a cast of characters determined to keep her heavy at all costs. "It's not my fault," she's saying. "In circumstances like these, how could *anyone* lose weight?"

This double message presents us with a dilemma. If we sympathize with her, and agree that she's a helpless victim, we're reinforcing her belief that she's destined to stay fat. Having sided with her belief that she can't change, the best we can offer is help in adjusting to her sad fate.

But there's a real problem with this approach: no client has ever asked us how to be fat and happy. Instead, no matter how victimized she feels, she seeks the magic formula that will cause her to lose weight.

We don't have a prayer of helping a woman who is overweight and overwhelmed unless we convince her to change her beliefs about her weight problem. She cannot allow helplessness to be her dominant emotion. And she cannot use the circumstances of her life, no matter how unfortunate, as excuses for her weight problem. As long as she thinks and feels like a victim, she'll act like one, and remain powerless over her body and her life. Only by accepting complete responsibility for her weight can she begin to change it.

By insisting that a woman stop thinking of herself as a victim, we aren't trying to convince her that her life is wonderful. All of our clients have difficult lives, and their problems certainly can't be solved just by wishing them away. But every woman can choose how she'll cope with her own circumstances. She can opt to let others direct her life or she can insist on retaining some measure of freedom and personal power. She can use this power to get sympathy and attention from others or she can use it to improve her life.

To persuade people to relinquish the victim role, we try to help them correct three basic misbeliefs. The first is the assumption that external conditions make weight problems *inevitable.* One or more of the following excuses are typical of those used to justify weight problems:

> "My parents always rewarded me with food when I was young."
> "I come from an ethnic family where eating is the center of activity."
> "I work in a bakery, so I'm constantly tempted."
> "I regularly have to entertain clients at restaurants."
> "My children want treats in the house at all times."
> "I have P.M.S., so I can't resist sweets at certain times of the month."
> "My husband . . . !"

We have no argument with claims that many factors contribute to a weight problem. But the connection is never inevitable. Obviously there are thin women whose parents used food to reward everything from good report cards to breathing out, and whose families celebrated every occasion, happy or sad, with a six course meal. Somehow they manage to overcome the influence of that family legacy. There are also women who work in bakeries without sampling all the goods; who don't mind eating a salad while clients indulge in elaborate meals; who buy their children treats that only a child could like; and who find ways to deal with P.M.S. without resorting to the very foods that make it worse. The inescapable conclusion is that thin is always a possibility, no matter what circumstances make fat seem the easier choice.

Does that mean that trying to determine the reasons for overeating is a waste of time? Not necessarily. The key here is the need to differentiate between an *explanation* and an *excuse*. An explanation provides some insight into the factors that contribute to a weight problem. Explanations can shed light on the circumstances that contribute to a problem, and they can be useful if they lead to insights that suggest a solution. For example, if a woman realizes that she breaks her diet every time she prepares a fattening treat for her children, she may decide to tell the children to fix their own snacks, or do without.

But it's more common for women to use these circumstances as excuses for their weight problems. They describe peculiarities of heredity or environment as if those circumstances not only explain their weight problem, but also make it unavoidable. They absolve themselves by placing the blame on external forces that no one could expect them to control.

This tendency to look for excuses is natural. Because overweight women are so often blamed for their condition, they try to convince themselves that it's not their fault they're fat. Then they can rightly expect sympathy instead of condemnation.

But excuses always make matters worse. Once responsibility for a weight problem is attributed to external forces, there's no hope of ever overcoming it. After all, if circumstances are beyond one's control, it's unreasonable to try to change them. All over-weight women can do is suffer. And eat. And suffer more.

So our first step in therapy is to convince our clients that even though circumstances may *contribute* to a weight problem, they don't *determine* the number on the scale. Genetic predisposition can make weight loss more difficult for some people, but they still can choose whether to be in the higher or lower end of their biological weight range. Children can certainly learn bad habits at an early age, but new habits can be learned as adults. Some jobs put food within easy reach, but one can take or refuse the bait. And both hormones and husbands can stimulate bad moods, but food isn't the only pacifier.

Once clients accept the notion that yielding to circumstance is a choice and not a necessity, they are apt to start blaming their "fat personalities." Using phrases like "I'm the kind of person who . . . ," they refer to a part of their nature they can neither identify nor control. That's when we face the next challenge: to free them from the mistaken belief that if bad circumstances aren't to blame, the fault lies within a deep and uncontrollable part of themselves.

Why do women think they're "driven" to act in predeter-mined ways? Again, this belief is understandable, though erro-neous. It's natural to base predictions of the future on experience in the past. So a woman with a history of failed weight-loss attempts is likely to expect continual failure in the future.

But our years as therapists have made us optimists about the flexibility of "personality" and the potential for great change. Negative behaviors often ascribed to "personality" are more likely the result of not knowing how to do things differently. With the proper motivation and guidance, nearly everyone is capable of major change. We've seen people set aside longstand-ing patterns of depression, anxiety, insecurity, and passivity, and learn to follow more productive paths.

To set the stage for change, we help a client take a new look at both her past and her future. We emphasize that no matter how it seemed at the time, her past actions were dictated by choice, not necessity. She is as free to choose a different future path as she is to continue familiar outdated patterns.

In his book *How People Change,* Allen Wheelis stresses the importance of taking a fresh look at the impact of the past on the future. He points out that there is no one *true* version of the past, but there are more and less useful ways to look at our personal histories. He emphasizes that "the way we understand the past is determined . . . by the future we desire."[7] If we want to excuse ourselves, we blame our troubles on forces beyond our control. If we want to change, however, we can decide to take responsibility, and understand that we always have some freedom to choose among alternatives.

Wheelis acknowledges that life circumstances can restrict freedom of choice. But the restriction is never total, so the person still has some say in designing the outcome. As Wheelis says, "A farmer must know the fence which bounds his land, but need not spend his life standing there, looking out, beating his fists on the rails; better he till his soil, think of what to grow, where to plant the fruit trees."[8] Similarly, every overweight woman can define her realm of freedom as widely as possible, and then work within it to design a future that is better than the past.

Once our clients are willing to take responsibility for both past and future behavior, a final mistaken belief must be challenged. This is the common misconception that having the power to decide is the same as deciding to lose weight.

In fact, not everyone should lose weight. As we've illustrated time and again, a woman's weight is often intimately connected to other issues in her life, particularly her self-esteem, her sexual feelings, and her marital satisfaction. Therefore, *any decision about what to weigh is also a decision about how to live.* Only a thorough and honest self-examination of the very personal meanings of food and fat can lead to goals that are both meaningful and realistic.

VI

Weighing the Options

To lose or not to lose? The answer isn't as obvious as it may seem. To decide intelligently whether weight loss is worth the effort, it's essential to evaluate both the personal significance of overeating and being overweight, and the potential rewards and hazards of the thin life.

The issue is particularly complex for women, because their feelings about their weight can color every other aspect of their lives. For some women, what they weigh is the primary determinant of how they live. So the decision to lose or not lose weight must be made with great care.

Drawing upon the experiences of a variety of women, we'll investigate the pros and cons of weight gain and weight loss. First we'll look at the range of problems commonly associated with being overweight, and we'll show how weight loss often leads to much more satisfying lives. Then we'll examine the other side of the coin, by reviewing the experiences of women who are happier when heavy. We'll also share some of the "nightmares" that can greet a woman who achieves her weight-loss dreams.

Describing every possible outcome may seem to create more confusion than it resolves, but we have a method in mind. We're convinced that many women who struggle with their weight come up against barriers that are unexpected, confusing, and ultimately defeating. If they knew what to expect at the outset, they could more accurately predict their future.

Based on a careful consideration of the potential risks and benefits, some women resign themselves to being overweight, and spare themselves the frustration of more failed diet attempts. Others delay trying to lose weight until they feel more capable of handling the potential problems. And some women, armed with new knowledge and determination, feel better equipped to persevere and succeed.

THE HIGH COST
OF BEING OVERWEIGHT

Kay is a woman with a mission. After gaining and then losing over 100 pounds, she feels she has an important story to share. When she heard about our study, she almost begged us to interview her. "I want to give people hope," she said. "I've been through it all. I know what it's like to be 100 pounds overweight, and I know how life can change when you reach a normal weight." Here's just part of Kay's description:

> Being fat is the pits. People treat you differently; they look down on you. They assume that no self-respecting person would let herself get so fat, so they're hardly inclined to get to know you. We live in a fat-hating society in which we're judged incompetent if we're fat. It's too bad, but it's a fact of life.
>
> I bought right into those attitudes, and I decided I had no right to impose myself on others. So I never went anywhere or did anything. Of course staying home made

me more bored and depressed, and my eating problem only got worse. I felt trapped and helpless.

By the time I reached my high weight, I had only one dress. That's all I needed, since the one thing I did was play the organ for church once a week. Even that was difficult—I loved the music, but I hated being seen in public. All week, I dreaded Sunday because I had to go out of the house. My self-image was zero.

I think back on those days and I get mad. Mad at all the people who made me feel so bad about myself; and mad at myself for accepting their negative judgments. But I couldn't fight the system and learn to accept myself as a fat woman. I had to lose weight before I could gain self-respect.

Prejudice against obesity is established at a very early age. Fat children are shunned by their peers, and this negative impact often persists into adulthood. During adolescence, weight is more of an issue for girls. Boys gain acceptance for a wide variety of achievements, but girls are judged primarily by their appearance. No matter what they do, they're likely to be rejected if they don't have the "right look." The social isolation of overweight teenage girls often makes them passive and insecure.

Emphasis on looking good leads many, perhaps most, girls to become preoccupied with their weight. One research team found that between the ninth and twelfth grades, an increasing number of girls think of themselves as too fat, even when their weight is well within normal limits by any objective standard.[9] Fear of fat is the teenage girl's constant companion.

Many girls are so afraid of obesity that they become bulemic or even anorexic, disorders that have reached epidemic proportions. Another reaction is to be so obsessed with dieting that food becomes irresistible simply because it's forbidden. The deprivation of dieting leads to episodes of binge eating, which eventually create the weight problems the diets were designed to avoid.

The prejudice against overweight people doesn't end with the teenage years, and females continue to be the focus of discrimination. Although overweight men may be accepted on the basis of intelligence, financial status, or professional achievement, overweight women are still judged primarily—even by other women —on their appearance.[10] If their weight problem is severe, they're also likely to suffer discrimination on the job.[11] Employers often believe that overweight applicants are less healthy, less diligent, or less intelligent than thin job applicants.

Women have also recounted the humiliation of being ignored in stores while salespeople turn their attention to shoppers who are easier to fit. And there's often more than a trace of condescension in the attitudes of strangers. It's hard to fight the feelings of inferiority that result from frequent exposure to such treatment.

Of course some overweight women may be so self-conscious that they see disapproval where none exists. Yet the similarity of details in many of the descriptions convince us that thin people do look down on anyone they consider too fat.

For example, overweight women always mention the particular discomfort they feel while eating in public. One of our clients still shudders when she recalls the time she was walking down the street eating a frozen yogurt cone, and a passing stranger reprimanded her with the comment, "You don't need that." Instead of feeling angry at the audacity of this man, she felt apologetic, wanting to explain that it was yogurt and not ice-cream!

This kind of guilt is typical. As a result, some women try to do all their eating in private. This allows them to avoid disapproving looks and comments. But it also intensifies their feelings of hurt, loneliness—and hunger.

Eventually, most obese women become so self-conscious about

their bodies that they try to hide not only from other people, but also from themselves. As one of our clients described it:

> I don't even like to look at my whole face. If I'm combing my hair, it's only my hair I see. If I use a mirror to put on lipstick, I hold it so close that I don't have to look at my fat cheeks. I never look at my naked body, and I'd rather walk out of the house without checking my clothes than see myself full length. And most of all, I will *NEVER* let *ANYONE* take my picture.

It's tragic to see how many women accept the belief that they're failures as human beings simply because they weigh too much. Psychologists call this kind of self-condemnation "identification with the aggressor." When an overweight woman identifies with the anti-fat values of society, she turns her anger inward, and berates herself for her failure to be what everyone expects her to be. With each failed diet attempt, she becomes more depressed and self-conscious. Eventually, she may seek protection by isolating herself from the real and imagined negative judgments of other people, including her husband and friends:

> I've gained almost 60 pounds since getting married, and I hate the way I look. Not only will I not go out, I won't even invite people to come to our home because I'm so embarrassed about my looks. At my request, my husband cancelled a birthday party for me, and I've cancelled several neighborhood get-togethers because I can't stand to be seen. I also refuse to go out with my husband, because I don't want people to feel sorry for him.

This woman puts herself in a real bind. Her isolation protects her from embarrassment, but it also gives her unlimited opportunity to wallow in her negative feelings. The more she isolates herself, the worse she feels, and the more she eats. This self-defeating cycle can be neverending. And as the woman above admits: "I'm sure my husband would like to throttle me because I have a one-track mind. I don't think about sex, children, work, or anything else. I only dwell on my weight and how terrible it makes me feel."

A woman's feelings about her weight can also make it more difficult for her to get out of a bad marriage. We received numerous letters from women who were extremely unhappy with their husbands, but felt unable to end their marriages. Of course, this situation is hardly unique to obese women, but obesity can be an additional handicap. We've already explained how husbands can use their wives' weight as an excuse to ignore them, to abuse them, and to justify their own vices. When the wife feels inadequate because of her weight, she's much more likely to tolerate a husband she might leave if she were more self-confident.

Of all the ways in which weight gain can destroy marital happiness, the erosion of sexual satisfaction is by far the most common. According to our survey respondents, womens' inhibitions about being seen or touched when they feel fat are at least as much of a problem as their husbands' diminished sexual interest.

Over three-fourths of the women in our study reported that weight gain makes them less comfortable about nudity. Like this woman, thousands expressed negative feelings about their bodies: "I'm so self-conscious about the way I look undressed that I never let my husband see me naked. And I will only have sex at night. My husband does shift work, so there are many times we could have sex during the day, but I always find ways to avoid it."

Not surprisingly, it's difficult for a woman to surrender herself to sexual passion while silently criticizing various parts of her body and wondering what her husband is thinking. That's probably why over half of our respondents reported less sexual satisfaction when they were heavier. And as sex became less enjoyable, desire also declined. Sexual intimacy became just another reminder of their dissatisfaction with their bodies and with themselves.

Sometimes, though less often than one might expect, husbands reinforce their wives' bad feelings. Over one-third of our respondents said sexual overtures from their husbands decreased as their weight increased. And some wives doubted the sincerity of husbands who stayed sexually interested despite their weight gain. One of the more extreme reactions was expressed by a woman who said: "I hate my body so much when I'm fat that I lose respect for my husband when he wants to touch me."

Indeed it seems that some husbands just can't win. When their overweight wives become depressed and angry, almost any action can be negatively interpreted. A husband's interest *or* disinterest can be used as an excuse for his wife to withdraw sexually and emotionally. This kind of reaction suggests how a woman's distress about her weight can raise the stress level of her marriage.

Naturally, as weight problems become more severe, so do the complications. Those who are extremely obese are forced to acknowledge that they can't fit comfortably into a world designed for thin people:

> When I visit friends, I have to carefully examine every chair. I choose the one that looks most sturdy, lower myself carefully, and pray that the chair doesn't creak, or worse yet, crack.
>
> In theatres I will only sit in the aisle seat, with my husband next to me. Otherwise I will spill over into the

neighboring seat and get hostile looks from a stranger. I've even walked out of movies without seeing the show because all the aisle seats were taken.

Then there are the problems of finding attractive fashions in larger sizes. Designers are finally beginning to realize that large women want to look nice too, but for years we have had to use specialty catalogues or learn how to sew if we wanted nice clothes. In many different ways, obese women get regular reminders that we just don't fit.

But of all the consequences of being overweight, the most serious is the one least mentioned. While every overweight person can enumerate the unhappy social and emotional effects of obesity, few acknowledge the potential damage their weight can have on their health.

Many illnesses are associated with being overweight, including diabetes and heart disease. All obesity-related conditions are disturbing, and some are incapacitating. A panel of experts advising the National Institute of Health has identified obesity as a "potential killer," and advised everyone over 20 percent overweight to reduce.[12] That includes approximately thirty-four million Americans—one-fifth of the adult population! When the physiological consequences are added to the negative social and psychological effects of being overweight, the argument for losing weight becomes a very strong one.

WHEN LOSING IS WINNING

The psychological benefits of weight loss usually appear even before other people notice the change in appearance. Women often start to feel better about themselves simply knowing they're headed in the right direction. Consider the impact of a 10-pound weight loss on this woman, who's still at 215:

> When I lose even a little weight, big changes occur. My grooming becomes a priority, so I take better care of my face, hair, nails, and clothes. I become more active, since I don't feel I have to find excuses to avoid being seen in public. And I prepare better meals for my family because I have more money to spend on their food when I don't buy so much food for myself.

Like the many others who express delight in even a small weight loss, this woman went on to describe how her life became more productive the moment she felt she'd established control over her eating.

The crucial change is not in the woman's weight *per se,* but rather in her attitude about herself. As soon as she has some evidence that she can control her eating, instead of being controlled *by* it, she starts to feel better about herself.

Dramatic changes in attitude can result from very small changes in behavior. One of our clients told us how she passed up a piece of birthday cake at an office party. This act of self-control led her to proclaim: "I've rejoined the human race!"

Once she believes she can control her eating, a woman realizes that she can control other areas of her life as well. She takes more risks, gets good results, and forms a more positive self-image, based on what she can do, not just on what she weighs. Notice the change in Kay, the woman who wanted to spread the word about the joys of the thin life:

> Now that I've lost 100 pounds, I've become much more self-assured. I've proven to others that I'm not a deadbeat and a failure, and I've proven to myself that I

can do anything I set my mind to. While I was losing weight, I got a decent job, I improved my relationship with my husband, and, best of all, I started to really like myself. I now feel that all things are possible—all doors are open to me!

This may sound too good to be true, but many women claim that weight loss, once begun, allowed their hopes to become a reality. When they look better and feel more confident, other people treat them with more respect and consideration. This makes it easier for them to ask for what they deserve, and to do what's necessary to reach desired goals.

The newfound approval isn't limited to that of strangers. Many women said husbands reacted to weight loss by showing increased respect, affection, and sexual interest. Six of our survey respondents used exactly the same phrase: "He treats me now the way he did when we were first married!" One woman said, "I get many unsolicited hugs and kisses. Now I've not only got a daddy for my kids, but a lover for me." And another, feeling better about her own body, spoke of greater affection: "We are by nature a touching couple. But how much easier it is for me to let him touch me when what he feels isn't fat!"

When women enjoy their bodies more, they think about them less. This frees them to redirect their attention to others, and husbands are the major beneficiaries. One of our clients described this change by saying, "When I weigh 20 pounds less, I stop thinking only about how bad I look, and start thinking much more about how my husband feels." This change in her attitude added new life to a marriage that had been stale for years.

For most women, the major improvements are in the sexual sphere. Many tell of enjoying more frequent, more active, and more satisfying sex with their husbands. Some women see the change as the direct result of their husbands being more attracted to a thinner body. For example: "When I was at my high weight, my husband actually threatened to leave me because he hated my fat. Now that I'm close to my goal weight, he can't keep his hands off me."

A majority of women, however, believe that changes in their attitudes were as important as the changes in their weight. Women reported greater sexual desire and less sexual inhibition when they felt better about their bodies. This accounts for the fact that almost 60 percent of the women in our study have sex more often, and enjoy it more, after they lose weight.

Many letters support our conviction that attitude is as important as body weight. Some were from the 40 percent of our sample who said their weight had no effect on their husbands' sexual interest, but it made all the difference in their own willingness to be sexual, as this excerpt indicates:

> My husband has always found me attractive. He once said he'd be happy to make love to me even if I was covered with mud! But when my weight is lower, I find that I think about sex more often and I'm more relaxed about making love. Somehow the need to get up early the next morning (so "no sex tonight!") is less critical when I weigh less. Intimate caresses are more enjoyable too, because they're not the intrusions they once seemed.

Other women report that their husbands respond sensually to the revitalized self-images that accompany their weight loss:

> After gaining 32 pounds after the birth of my third child, I withdrew from my husband and he withdrew from me. Since losing this weight, I found a new me inside, and I liked what I found. Because I like myself better, I can give myself more fully to my husband, and

in return he is much more responsive to me. As a result, we're enjoying each other more than we ever did before —both in and out of bed.

This woman was one of many who realized that her improved self-image was partly responsible for the improvements in her sex life. Since the psychological component of sex is at least as important as the physical one, it takes more than a slimmer body to reignite passion.

The improved self-esteem that accompanies weight loss changes the meaning of sex for some women. It frees them from using sex as a means of confirming their own desirability:

At my heaviest, sex was *urgent* because it was the only time I felt loved or needed. Even though I was too fat to participate actively when I weighed 211 pounds, I had to have the closeness. At 145, I'm more mobile, I feel better about being seen in the nude, and I enjoy taking baths with my husband. And best of all, we make love now because *we* want to, not because *I* have to.

As a woman finds increased emotional and sexual intimacy with her husband, food often becomes less important. Having overcome the emotional emptiness of a burned-out relationship, she has no need to seek out edible substitutes for love and affection. One woman describes how her husband's attention is a perfectly satisfying replacement for overeating: "I don't worry about maintaining my weight loss—the extra affection I get from my husband provides all the motivation I need. I've discovered that I'm happier enjoying his approval and having my ego restored than I ever was with an entire chocolate-cream pie."

Of course weight loss doesn't always increase a woman's marital and sexual satisfaction. When her marriage is very unhappy, weight loss can't begin to solve all of her problems. And if her husband has his own reasons for wanting his wife to stay fat, weight loss is sure to make matters worse. On the other hand, if she wants to end her marriage, losing weight can only help. One woman offered a striking example of how her weight loss gave her the confidence to liberate herself from a destructive relationship:

> My first husband beat me up twice while we were dating. Both times he was drunk and jealous about my dating other men, so I figured it would stop when we were married. What a jerk I was! He stopped being a "gentleman" when I became his wife, and he started hitting me drunk or sober when I didn't do things exactly his way. I was too embarrassed to tell my family or friends, so I isolated myself from people and consoled myself with food. After I lost three friends and gained 30 pounds, I realized I was so boring, depressed, and ugly that I would hit me too. That's when I hit bottom.
>
> He worked days so I took a swing-shift job. He used the money I earned to buy liquor, but I used the job to buy time. In six months I weighed 12 pounds *less* than I did when we were married. That's when I got the nerve to deliver an ultimatum: "Hit me one more time and you won't have the time to say goodbye!" He managed to control himself for a few days before he pushed me down the front steps hard enough to break my wrist. I never even went back into the house for my clothes. (Most of them were too big anyway!) I divorced him and I'm now married to a wonderfully loving and considerate man. I owe my new life and my new husband to losing 42 pounds.

Obviously, weight loss alone can't guarantee a "new life." But the increased self-confidence that accompanies it often helps

women to design lives that are far more satisfying. And given the
health benefits of having a trimmer body, the happier life can be
a longer one too!

WHEN WEIGHT LOSS LEADS
TO TROUBLE

Losing weight does not guarantee happiness; for many it brings
on an array of unanticipated problems. A very vocal minority of
women in our study were so deeply disappointed with the after-
effects of weight loss that they wished they had never lost a
pound. Although their experiences are exceptions to the rule,
they provide a sobering reminder that a thin life isn't necessarily
a happy one. Since losing weight is often a major ordeal, no one
should undertake a reducing program without being aware of
some of the possible negative consequences.

We've already described the threat of increased sexual attractiveness, and how being the object of sexual attention can be just
as anxiety-provoking as being overweight and ignored. A few
working women also described the aggravation of being judged
too attractive to be competent. These women discovered that just
as some people assume fat women are dumb, others assume pretty
women can't be intelligent or dedicated to their careers. They
expected their weight loss to lead to greater acceptance; instead
they found they had to work twice as hard to prove their worth:

> I've been a CPA for 12 years, and from the beginning
> I was well liked in the firm. Two years ago, I lost a lot
> of weight, and soon after I received a major promotion.
> Almost immediately, people I thought of as friends
> started keeping their distance. One day I heard two of my
> coworkers—a man and a woman—speculating that I'd

been promoted because my boss was interested in me. I was hurt by their gossip and infuriated that they couldn't overlook the weight loss and recognize my competence.

As this woman learned, both men and women can react negatively to a woman's weight loss and her new attractiveness. Some women find that friendships with other women deteriorate when they lose weight. Generally, these problems are the result of jealousy:

> I never thought I would lose my closest friend when I lost 25 pounds, but that's exactly what happened. As long as we experimented with the same diets and joked about our weight-loss struggles, we had a great time together. But once I found a program I could stick with, she was "too busy to talk" when I called, "just about to go out" when I dropped in, and always had "a thousand things to do" when I suggested we meet for lunch.
>
> I'm deeply hurt by her rejection. We had been friends since the eighth grade. How could she let all that go just because I lost weight? Could she be that jealous?

Jealousy is one possibility; personal insecurity is another. People often compare themselves to their friends, and when the comparisons are unfavorable, they may try to counter feelings of inadequacy by terminating the friendships.

If relationships aren't ended, they may be peppered with subtle, stinging indications of disapproval. Some of our clients have described the edge in the voice of other women who say: "My, you've lost so much weight! Don't you worry about being too thin?" Others were accused of being too self-absorbed or selfish, subjected to snide statements like: "It must be nice to have the time to pay so much attention to your weight." Such comments are seldom enough to cause a woman to regain her lost weight, but certainly can take some of the pleasure out of the accomplishment.

Problems also arise when a newly thin friend's attractiveness becomes a threat. Wary about her potential appeal, some women move away from, or even sever friendships. As one woman who was relegated to the status of former friend wrote:

> I used to walk every morning with three friends in the neighborhood. And we'd often have barbecues or parties with our husbands on weekends. Our exercise routine worked better for me than for the others, and only I lost weight. I was proud of my weight loss, but my friends seemed jealous. One of them even told me she didn't want her husband to see me in a bathing suit. I thought she was joking, but soon after the jealous remarks started, the weekend gatherings stopped. I can't believe that my friends would think I'd have any interest in their husbands!

Another set of problems can evolve from the positive psychological changes that accompany weight loss. A major weight reduction is usually the catalyst for a kind of "rebirth," from which a woman emerges not only thinner, but also more confident and more assertive. But her husband, family, and friends have not been similarly transformed, and these people may not be pleased with the changes they see. It's as if the formerly fat woman walks onto the stage with a new costume and new set of lines, while all the other actors are in their old garb with their old scripts, ready to go on with the drama as traditionally performed.

As a result, the formerly fat woman may not feel comfortable with some of her old relationships. There are those who liked her better when she was insecure and willing to do almost anything to be accepted. In her "former life," she may have eagerly complied with the wishes of others, even when those wishes were unreasonable. Once she gains self-assurance, she'll likely refuse unreasonable or undesirable requests. This can destabilize relationships in which she was valued more for what she did than for who she was.

As we've said, weight losses don't have to be dramatic to create major psychological changes. This was poignantly illustrated by a couple we saw for marriage therapy. Roy and Sarah had been married for eleven years. They met the day they started college, and they married at the end of their junior year. Roy wanted to be a doctor, and Sarah supported him through his medical training. As soon as he finished his internship, they started a family, and after their second child was born, Sarah quit her job and stayed home to care for the children.

Because Roy had chosen a demanding specialty, he was away from home most of the time, leaving Sarah in charge of all family matters. Even when he was home, he was too tired to participate in family life. Still, Sarah never complained. As she described it: "I was content to be a doctor's wife and a mother."

When Sarah turned 30, she started to take a greater interest in her health. She joined an athletic club, started cooking nutritious meals, and eliminated additives and preservatives from her diet. As an unexpected benefit of these changes, she lost 26 pounds. According to Roy, Sarah looked better than she did when they first met. Unfortunately for Roy, Sarah's expectations changed with her weight. This is how she described it:

> The "new me" expects more excitement. Maybe it's because I feel better about myself, maybe it's because of the compliments I receive. Whatever the reason, I want to do different things with Roy on every level. I want

him to be home more, so we can have more time to talk. I want to escape with him for romantic weekends and holidays. I want to spruce up our sex life, and get out of our boring routine. Roy tells me he's satisfied with the way things have always been. But the old ways are no longer good enough for me!

Husbands like Roy often feel betrayed by the changes their wives have made. Especially when men have intentionally chosen women who were compliant, they may resent demands to change the unwritten rules that governed their marriage. When the wives start to make demands, and husbands are bewildered, the relationships may be strained to the point of dissolution.

What kinds of demands are made by thinner, more confident wives? Like Sarah, many want more romance. This is translated into requests for time, talk, and affection. And when weight loss has given a woman the confidence to work outside the home, she'll usually want her husband to take on more responsibility for child care and housework. She may also want more say in how the family finances are handled, especially when she is directly contributing to the family income. If the husband doesn't cooperate, battle lines will be drawn.

Whether or not she makes the transition from housewife to paid employee, a woman's weight loss can increase her sense of independence. As she becomes more confident, her husband may fear that she no longer needs him, and worry that soon she will no longer want him:

My husband was extremely loving, considerate, and kind when I was fat. Now that I've lost a lot of weight, he's none of these things. I have become a very strong, self-sufficient person who is independent in all ways. He was more comfortable when I was unsure of myself and depended on him for everything.

In extreme cases, a husband's insecurity can drive him to end the marriage. Here's just one story of a marriage that ended when the husband couldn't cope with his wife's independence:

> When I lost 47 pounds, my husband said I had never been so pretty. But while he enjoyed my improved disposition, he went crazy worrying that my new size would make me "unmanageable." He had gotten used to my being home all the time, and didn't want to take the risk that I might decide I could do just as well without him. He became depressed, started to drink, and eventually ended a 16-year marriage.

Of course, we didn't have an opportunity to hear this husband's side of the story, and we must assume that the situation was more complex than it appears. Still, it shows how weight loss can trigger a chain reaction that can not only destabilize a marriage, but ultimately destroy it.

The most common marital problem resulting from a wife's weight loss is her husband's jealousy. As we've already emphasized, some husbands want to keep their wives fat to assure their fidelity. When the wife of an insecure husband loses weight, her husband may have trouble managing his suspicions and fears. He may "cope" by withdrawing from her, by becoming abusive, or by having affairs.

The appeasement of a jealous husband is not a compelling reason to stay fat. In our opinion, any relationship that is dependent upon one partner's obesity and lack of self-esteem is not worth saving. But some women are determined to stay married no matter what the emotional cost. They're the ones who may be forced to decide whether being thin is worth the price. The decision may be reduced to the choice between accepting a husbands' insecurity about having a thin wife, or their own insecurity about being a fat wife.

When a woman's weight loss disrupts the balance in a marriage, the negative effects almost always show up in the bedroom. Husbands and wives both contribute to the problem, and both suffer as a result. Wives who feel their weight loss makes them "superior" to husbands who are still overweight may decide that their husbands are sexually unappealing. Anticipating this reaction, some husbands withdraw from sex before their wives have a chance to reject them.

Dieting can also disrupt a woman's sex life. A weight-loss regimen often means intent focus on menus, measured food intake, exercise routines, and small bodily changes. As one woman put it:

> In successful dieting, one is very efficient, completely under control, and somewhat selfish. This leads to an independent feeling and what my husband calls my "businesslike mode." It has been very difficult for me to switch to a more relaxed mode—particularly a sexual one. My husband and I had an affectionate, active sex life when I was heavy. Now our lovemaking is easier physically, but much less satisfying. Most of the time I'd rather go to sleep.

This reaction is understandable when one considers the vigilance required to lose weight by strict dieting. When a woman feels she must never let down her guard, it's very difficult to relax, even while making love. Thus, the dieting "mindset," while fostering independence and self-control, can potentially interfere with intimacy.

Then there are women who resent their husbands' increased interest after weight loss. They are insulted by what they see as a lustful, impersonal reaction to their thinner bodies. A woman who resents her husband's increased sexual interest usually harbors deep resentment of his disinterest when she was heavy. The feelings of rejection are not forgotten, and weight loss gives a woman the courage to express some of the anger that existed when she was heavier and less confident.

Naturally, a husband will be confused by his wife's anger at what he probably feels is the highest compliment. Part of the problem may be due to a common (though not universal) sex difference; men are more likely to respond to the physical aspects of sexuality, while women put more value on its emotional aspects. This would explain a wife's anger at her husband's seeming inability to look beyond the surface, and her husband's confusion over this expectation.

In general, post weight-loss disappointments stem from a woman's mistaken belief that fat is at the root of all her problems, and that having a thin body will improve every aspect of her life. Although it seems obvious that weight loss can't solve problems that aren't weight-related, many women who struggle to become thin are crushed when they discover that their marriages are still faulty, or their sex lives still unfulfilling. They pin their hopes on weight loss as a cure-all, and they're naturally disappointed when weight loss fails to provide total relief.

There's one more disappointment that can confront women who lose a great amount of weight; a few find that they actually look worse. Some women discovered wrinkles that were not so noticeable before, others were distressed to find that their breasts had shrunk; and another group was aware of stretch marks and loose skin. As one woman said: "Ugly wasn't what I expected when I lost weight, and I feel cheated and even conned by those who promised a wonderful life at goal weight."

Much worse than these visual changes were the chronic physical ailments described by women who had subjected themselves to surgical procedures or radical dieting to lose weight. Complications due to side effects of extreme weight loss methods caused more than one woman to wonder if she had made the right choice.

In summary, the rewards of losing weight can be offset by a number of negative consequences. Some of the problems may be due to expecting more than weight loss can deliver. But the majority of problems relate to the dramatic improvements in self-esteem that accompany weight loss. As a woman begins to assert herself, relatives and friends have to adjust to the "new woman," or she must return to her old heavy self to restore the balance. Assuming that no woman wants to regress, one of the hidden costs of losing weight is the need to help other people to accept the changes that she worked so hard to achieve.

CHOOSE NOT TO LOSE?

Should anyone decide to stay fat? Maybe so. We think three categories of women could benefit from focusing on self-acceptance rather than losing weight:

1. *Women who aren't ready to give up the security of being overweight.* Fat provides them with the protection they feel is essential to their peace of mind.
2. *Women who are extremely distressed over small amounts of excess weight.* They see themselves as obese, and experience many of the psychological disadvantages of being fat. But

more objective observers would agree that the problem is truly "all in their heads."

3. *Women for whom weight control is a full-time, stressful job.* They may sincerely prefer to be thin, but the singleminded pursuit of that goal demands too much attention. They are left with little time and energy for other people and activities.

The stories of women who are torn between wanting and fearing weight loss have turned up throughout our book. Some stay fat to keep their marriages intact. Past experience with weight loss has convinced them that their marriages could not withstand the dramatic changes in appearance or confidence. Others feel there's a connection between fat and fidelity—fat protects them from the possibility of extramarital affairs. And some feel their extra weight is armor against physical attack. Being larger, they maintain, helps them to appear and feel less vulnerable. Finally, there are women who find that men treat them more respectfully when they're heavier and not being viewed as sex objects.

Some people would argue that these reasons are not compelling enough to justify staying fat. But we disagree. If a woman is convinced of the benefits of her excess weight, she won't stay thin for long. Losing weight is difficult, and being thin brings its own stresses. If a woman has equally compelling reasons for being thin or being heavy, she'll opt for staying overweight because it's easier.

In principle, all women can develop the skills they need to cope with weight loss. Some can do it on their own while others need the help of support groups. But when the underlying fears are of long duration and are not well understood, they are best handled with competent professional help.

If the needed help isn't available, it doesn't make sense for women to spend their lives vacillating between higher "safer" weights and lower threatening weights. For one thing, the constant yo-yo of weight loss and gain is likely to be more physically harmful than maintaining a steadier higher weight. And for women who are ambivalent about being thin, continual weight fluctuations take a heavy psychological toll.

There's no permanent way out until the underlying feelings of inadequacy are confronted and overcome. So until these fears are conquered, staying overweight may be the best alternative.

The second group of women have weight problems that are mostly "in their heads." These women are within twenty percent of their recommended weights, so weight poses few if any health risks. Nor does weight interfere with their social lives, careers, or marriages. But their self-esteem is almost completely dependent upon being thin, and their preoccupation with weight may be all-consuming. Generally, as their weight goes up, their self-esteem goes down.

Equating thinness with self-worth can lead a woman to condemn herself for even the slightest weight gain. She ignores the fact that even a very slim woman can pinch a bit of fat that is doing her no harm. Rage and depression can be brought on by a tiny bulge that no one else would notice. Here's one of the many letters we received describing the impact of infinitesimal variations in weight:

> I'm embarrassed about the way my body looks, and I spend my whole life going up and down emotionally according to how much I weigh and how many compliments I receive from other people. When I gain two pounds, I pound the flab on my legs and am filled with self-hatred.
>
> As soon as I wake up each morning, I get on the scale. If I've lost weight, the day's a winner. If I've stayed the

same, I know I'll have an average day. But if I've gained
weight, I will be miserable all day long, and I won't be
able to relax until I get rid of those ugly pounds.

In their desperation to meet unrealistically low weight loss
goals, women may turn to bizarre diets or dangerous drugs. We
heard from women who tried eating nothing but grapefruit or
lettuce, and others who became dependent on amphetamines.
Obsession with weight can reach the point of fanaticism where
ties to reality become fragile. We heard from a woman who lost
30 pounds to reach her goal weight, but then decided she was still
far too fat, so she kept on losing: "Now I'm near what I consider
to be my perfect weight, and though other people tell me I look
sick, I think they're just jealous. I need to get down to 85 pounds.
I know that sounds low, but I have very light bones. When I
weigh over 90, I'm too visible no matter where I go." Obviously
this woman is now anorexic, but she wasn't always that way. Her
story illustrates the danger of becoming so obsessed with weight
loss that it becomes impossible to be thin enough.

Even a less extreme preoccupation can lead otherwise sensible
women to unreasonable behavior. They may stock up on over-
priced, overprocessed, and undernutritious foods simply because
the foods are labeled "diet." These women scan bookshelves and
magazine racks for the magical shortcut to easy and permanent
weight loss. They take appetite suppressants, and when they give
in to their urges to overeat, they purge.

None of these approaches is remotely related to healthy and
permanent weight loss. Methods like these have failed time and
time again, and should be abandoned. We firmly believe "If at
first you don't succeed, try something else."

One suggested "something else" is forgetting about weight loss
goals that are too low and unrealistic. The typical female pattern
of fat distribution includes some curves that are not found on

models with figures like adolescent boys. Some of this fat cannot —and should not—be eliminated. Unrealistic expectations only sentence a woman to unnecessary feelings of inadequacy. As one woman wrote: "I feel reasonably comfortable with my weight. I don't have a bulging stomach, and I can still count my chins on one finger. Since I'm not so bad objectively, it's a pity that I feel so inadequate when I compare myself to the standard the media sets for women."

We suggest that women who have spent years battling an extra five to fifteen pounds might consider conceding, and turning their attention to different, more attainable goals that have nothing to do with weight. This is especially true for women who use minor weight "problems" to avoid coming to grips with more pressing issues. We've seen clients who have severe marital problems, difficulties with delinquent children, and even life-threatening illnesses, yet who seek therapy for losing weight. When weight is clearly a smokescreen, women are infinitely better off forgetting about weight and concentrating on other issues.

A final group of women should consider abandoning weight loss efforts: those whose weight maintenance depends on an intolerable level of deprivation. They have lost weight time and time again, but they can only maintain their losses by continuous stringent dieting. Even with regular vigorous exercise, they have tremendous difficulty maintaining their goal weights.

These women have bodies that don't naturally conform to current standards of thinness. What is considered "normal" eating for other people is overeating for them, and only by "undereating" can they stay anywhere close to slim. We suggest that if their weight remains in the medically safe range (less than twenty percent overweight), they should ask themselves if the rewards of being thin are worth the high cost of achieving and maintaining a lower weight.

There isn't one right answer to this question. For some women, being thin is so important that it's worth the effort, even if weight maintenance is an all-consuming task. We know women who spend their lives being hungry and willingly accepting the feeling of deprivation. But for others, the price is too high. Food is a major pleasure that they're unwilling to forgo, even though it means having a body that falls short of the ideal.

Other women for whom low weights are unrealistic are those with physical problems that complicate the already difficult process of weight loss. Some have injuries or chronic conditions that make exercise difficult or impossible: for example, arthritis in ankles and knees may make even walking arduous.

Certain medical conditions require the avoidance of many foods that comprise a well-balanced, reduced calorie diet. For example, people with diverticulitis who have to avoid high fiber foods may not be able to lose weight without further health damage. They may also need medication that interferes with weight loss. For them, dieting only compounds preexisting medical problems.

Is it realistic to expect women to accept themselves at higher weights and ignore social pressures to be thin? Though difficult, it can be done. Members of the National Association to Aid Fat Americans, a nationwide support group for fat people, believe that self-torture directed toward an impossible ideal is sheer foolishness. They not only accept their large size, they take pride in it. Some are even delighted with weights ranging from 200 to 400 or more pounds.

The key here is a sense of self worth based on factors other than weight. Every one of these fat women refuses to go along with society's attempts to make her feel inadequate because of her size. A 440-pound woman described how she learned to accept her weight and thereby accept herself:

> I'm different from most other people because I'm bigger than they are. But I want the same things they do,

and I'm hurt by the things that hurt them. I stopped looking at my size as something to be ashamed of and started looking at it as my uniqueness. I'm special—and I have many assets. Instead of fretting about what I weigh, I focus on what I can do in life. Now my self-image is that of a big, accomplished, unique woman.

Once these women appreciate themselves, their bodies become a valuable part of a worthy person. And once they accept their bodies, they are no longer self-conscious. In contrast to the many women who let their inhibitions about their weight ruin their sex lives, these women usually have very satisfying sexual experiences:

The important thing is to accept your size and become more comfortable with your own sexuality. You must listen to yourself, to the feelings that come from inside you. I agree with the person who said "size is an attitude." The same is true with sexuality. You have to believe that you can be a warm, loving, sensual, giving person. Once you believe this, your sexuality will unfold.

Two factors seem important in achieving this level of self-acceptance: the interest of a loving man who appreciates a large woman, and the support of a group of like-minded people. The group serves as a microsociety that not only accepts, but often prefers, women of above-average weight. And it allows them a feeling of belonging that they seldom find in their daily lives.

These women illustrate an important point. They are committed to the idea that it's not necessary to conform to common standards of beauty in order to accept oneself and be accepted by others. They believe that the major source of unhappiness among fat women is not their fat, but their lack of self-esteem. And they prove that self-esteem can be improved *without* losing weight. Whether they see fat as beautiful, or merely irrelevant, they don't let society's ideas about the "ideal" shape affect their feelings about themselves.

While we agree that beauty is in the eye of the beholder, we can't ignore the negative health effects of obesity. Therefore, being extremely obese is not our prescription for a happy life. But these women provide very positive examples for others who allow their lives to be ruined by obesity they can't control. There are tremendous benefits to redirecting attention from weight to attitude. If the only reasonable choice is between being "fat and miserable" or "fat and happy," why be miserable?

VII

Making the Decision

Since every woman is unique, each must decide for herself whether or not to make yet another weight loss attempt. We help our clients structure the choice by posing the following questions.

MAINTAINING YOUR PRESENT WEIGHT

Physical Aspects
1. Has your doctor told you it is safe for you to maintain your present weight?
2. Does weight loss create health problems for you because you frequently lose and then regain 10 or more pounds?
3. Are you less than 20 percent above your ideal weight?

If you answered "yes" to all of the above, *it may be medically safe* for you to stay at your present weight.

Psychological Aspects
1. Do you basically like yourself as you are?
2. Do you find that weight loss requires a great effort that leaves you frustrated and depressed?

3. Are you afraid of being more vulnerable to unwanted sexual advances as a consequence of weight loss?
4. Is not reaching goal weight even more depressing than being overweight?
5. Is eating your major source of satisfaction?
6. Are you unwilling to exercise?

If you answered "yes" to at least two of the questions above, *it may be psychologically advisable* for you to maintain your present weight.

Social Aspects
1. Are you as interested in employment opportunities when you're overweight as you are when you weigh less?
2. Do you participate in as many recreational activities when you're overweight as you do when you weigh less?
3. Do you socialize as easily when you weigh more as you do when you weigh less?
4. Do you feel that people like you as well when you're overweight as they do when you weigh less?

If you answered "yes" to all of the questions above, *it may be socially advisable* for you to stay at your present weight.

EFFECTS OF LOSING WEIGHT

Physical Aspects
1. Has your doctor advised you to lose weight?
2. Have you *ever* been told that you have diabetes, hypertension, or other weight-exacerbated diseases?
3. Do you become easily exhausted climbing stairs, walking a few blocks, or making love?

4. Are you 30 percent or more above your recommended weight?

If you answered "yes" to any of the questions above, *it is medically important* for you to lose weight.

Psychological Aspects
1. Do you regularly feel depressed about being overweight?
2. Are you are inhibited from doing things you enjoy because you're self-conscious about your weight?
3. Do your thoughts about your weight interfere with your involvement with other people, activities, work, etc.?
4. Is fear of failing one of your major reasons for not trying to lose weight?

If you answered "yes" to any of the questions above, *it may be psychologically desirable* for you to lose weight.

Social Aspects
1. Do you believe your weight affects your marriage in a negative way?
2. Do you believe your weight interferes with your professional opportunities?
3. Would weight loss greatly increase your social opportunities?

If you answered "yes" to any of the questions above, *it may be socially desirable* for you to lose weight.

The answers to these questions may not lead to an obvious decision; they're intended only to point the way to a wise choice. In considering the answers, pay particular attention to the items that are most relevant. And try to think of other issues these questions don't address.

To illustrate how some women made their decisions, we'll offer a few examples from our clinical files, starting with Marian, a 37-year-old woman who weighed 182 pounds. She felt her 40 pound weight gain was directly related to her marriage, which started to go sour soon after the wedding, nine years earlier. Her husband, an alcoholic, was a great complainer—about her family, her housekeeping, and especially her weight. What little extra money they had, he spent on alcohol, which he drank with his buddies at a downtown bar. Still, Marian said she loved her husband and believed she could make the marriage work.

Marian told herself that no man would tolerate a wife as fat and ugly as she felt she was, and until she lost weight, she had no right to demand that her husband clean up his act. But she couldn't stick to a diet because she depended on food for comfort.

Marian's major reason for attempting to lose was to try to make her marriage better. But we felt her attention was misdirected. Although weight loss might improve her self-esteem, it would not turn her husband into a new man. After all, their problems started before she was fat, and her weight was much more likely to be a symptom than a cause of her unhappy marriage.

We recommended that Marian seek counseling with her husband for their marital problems. If he refused to go, individual counseling could help her raise her self-esteem. Until she felt better about herself and her situation, her weight loss attempts were likely to fail.

Another client, Doreen, was only mildly overweight, but she felt much happier and more confident when she weighed 15 pounds less. At the same time, she was close to accepting her extra weight as a necessary cushion against extramarital sex. When she compared the advantage of feeling better about her body to the disadvantage of risking an affair and a marital breakup, she decided she'd rather keep her extra weight. We agreed that given those two alternatives, she might be healthier and happier by accepting herself with the 15 extra pounds.

But we also pointed out that there was an alternative she hadn't considered. The fact that she was tempted to go to bed with other men didn't mean she was destined to have extramarital sex. She could learn to accept her feelings of attraction, without thinking she had to act on them. She could cultivate a new outlook that would allow her to enjoy looking her best, without having to worry about it.

Finally, we have a tragic story to tell. Sue was one of our clients whose warmth and wit made it a joy to spend time with her. We wondered at times if we shouldn't pay her for the hours we spent together because they were such pleasant times. Unfortunately, her obesity had already led to severe diabetes-related circulatory and visual problems. In addition, her weight prevented her from being able to have surgery she needed to improve her health.

Unfortunately, even these threats paled next to the pleasure Sue found in overeating. She truly believed that the immediate rush she got from eating was too great to pass up for the delayed gratification of better health. So despite the urging of her family, her final decision was to keep her extra weight and hope for the best.

Sue's case reminded us that we can't control the outcome of anyone else's decision. Weight loss is an individual undertaking, and the motivation to do it must come from within. We can point out the costs and benefits, and we can recommend the approach most likely to succeed, but we have neither the power nor the right to make the final decision for anyone else. With this in mind, all we can do is urge extreme care in contemplating the costs and benefits of losing weight . . . or deciding not to lose.

It may help to keep in mind some of the guidelines we use with the women we treat:

1. *Never try to use weight loss to solve problems that are not weight-related.* Weight loss is as likely to create new difficulties as it is to resolve old ones.
2. *If you have fears about the consequences of weight loss, try to confront and conquer the fears before trying to lose weight.*
3. *If you are only a little overweight, and weight loss poses a major challenge to you, you may want to work on learning to accept yourself as you are and forget about your weight.*
4. *If being overweight poses an immediate, major health risk, losing weight is always worth the effort, no matter how much effort it takes.* As anyone who has been seriously ill can attest, without health you have nothing.

Remember that no decision has to be permanent. Experience always brings additional knowledge which may in turn influence subsequent decisions. As we've pointed out, it often makes sense to accept extra weight temporarily, while dealing with some of the obstacles to weight loss. At that point, a reevaluation will be in order, and a new strategy may emerge.

VIII

Getting Ready
to Lose Weight

Three broken chocolate chip cookies are left in the bottom of the bag. An overweight woman, feeling overwhelmed by all the things that have gone wrong throughout the day, is as likely to pass up those cookies as she is to tear up a winning ticket in a million-dollar lottery. She's in emotional turmoil, and she is desperately seeking some relief. The need is in her head. But she'll respond by trying to fill her stomach.

If this woman belonged to the typical weight control program, she'd probably be chided for having cookies in the house, and she'd definitely be urged to resist the temptation to overeat. In response to the reprimands, she might find the "willpower" to stick to her diet for a week or two. But eventually she'd return to her old habits, because her need to overeat hasn't been addressed, merely repressed.

The common approach to dealing with overeating "directly" by prescribing diet and exercise has only recently been challenged. Research is just beginning to catch up with what overweight women have known for years: diets fail because they don't consider the important psychological benefits of food and fat. Because many aspects of women's lives are influenced by their overweight, they must be ready to assume the risks of the thin life before they can succeed in losing weight. And because most women who overeat have compelling reasons for doing so, their eating urges must be controlled if their weight loss is to be permanent.

The single most important lesson we've learned from our combined thirty years of work with overweight women is that no woman succeeds in losing weight until she's ready. For most women, being "ready" requires two major changes:

1. *They must feel certain that being thin is more beneficial than being fat;*
2. *They must put food in its proper role by learning how to eat to live, rather than living to eat.*

Making these changes is seldom easy. As we've already seen, overweight can offer the following benefits:

- protection from sexual threats;
- protection against extramarital sex;
- a means of expressing (or repressing) anger;
- protection against the risk of failure.

When the advantages of being overweight are stronger than the bad effects, weight-loss attempts will be half-hearted at best.

Like fat, food plays an important role in the lives of many married women. Let's briefly review the four major patterns of overeating that so often lead to extra inches.

Casual eaters are happy with their marriages. They don't use food as an emotional crutch; they overeat for sheer enjoyment.

Eating may be the major pleasure these women share with their husbands. They usually go out to eat quite regularly, and they like to entertain together.

Because they seldom binge, casual eaters may gain weight slowly. But if they shun exercise, the accumulated weight gains of five or more pounds each year will do major damage over time.

Bored eaters also may have satisfying marriages. They attribute their eating problems to circumstances beyond their control, but their husbands are seldom seen as villains.

The typical bored eater is the housewife/mother who has limited variety in her daily routine. She spends most of her time engaged in tasks that are crucial, but lacking in excitement or intellectual challenge.

For the bored eater, eating can help spice up a dull routine. But while food is a major source of diversion and pleasure, it's not the woman's sole resource. Eating is an end-in-itself that rescues her from the tedium of the hour. Unfortunately, its observable effects are proportionate to its use, and the pounds can add up with alarming speed.

Sensual eaters usually have serious complaints about their marriages. They may be disappointed by routine or nonexistent sex lives, or by relationships lacking affection and intimacy. Wives in these frustrating relationships live with a general sense of deprivation that they try to compensate for by eating. Food becomes a substitute for the "real thing."

Sensual eaters are in for significant weight gain, since the desire for intimacy is seldom outgrown. Their emotional hunger may gradually be buried beneath an ever-increasing hunger for food.

Coping eaters face more extreme situations. They are unhappy with their marriages and are often besieged by self-doubts. Some are victims of physical abuse; others are emotionally abused or neglected to the point of chronic anxiety and depression.

Food means sanity for these women. When a marriage can hardly be endured, and when self-esteem is almost nil, the pleasure of eating may feel like the key to emotional survival.

Bored, sensual, and coping eaters initially turn to food for specific kinds of emotional satisfaction. But once overeating is well-established, it usually becomes a psychological symptom that emerges in response to any and every problem. Allen Wheelis describes a symptom as:

> not the expression of a specific conflict, but a response to any conflict, any tension, a way of running from whatever seems too much; it has become a mode of being in the world. The patient may feel it as alien, want to be rid of it, but it has become useful in a thousand unnoticed ways; its removal would not be simple relief but would expose the patient to conflicts which he has no other way of handling.[13]

Based on the assumption that overeating is often a symptom of other problems, *we never start obesity treatment by telling people to eat less.* Rather, we start by helping them find other ways to satisfy their psychological hunger. That means we must find out why they overeat, and then work on changes that diminish their desire.

When we first see an overweight client, we ask her to keep two records for a week. On one, she keeps track of the times she thought about her weight. We ask her where she was, what she was doing, and whether she felt good or bad about her body.

The other record is an eating diary in which she records not only what, when, and where she eats, but also how she was feeling before and after she ate. In addition, she is asked to note any ideas about what led to her feelings. This provides important information about the factors that typically lead to overeating.

Once we have a fix on a woman's circumstances, beliefs, and feelings, we determine where productive changes can be made. Then we encourage her to make those changes *before* working on weight loss. By asking her to reduce her stress level and start feeling better about herself before she changes her eating habits, we're helping her make overeating and overweight less necessary. Once she feels more in control of her life and emotions, it's much easier to develop the energy, patience, and optimism necessary for successful weight loss.

Let's look at an example of how this philosophy is applied. Val was a client of ours who defined herself as a coping eater. The stresses in her life were not unusual, but they were no less difficult for being common. She had a hyperactive son she couldn't control, a demanding husband she felt unable to please, and long days full of demanding work, including the care of an ailing mother. Val wasn't sure she could manage without the comfort of her favorite foods. Unfortunately, her negative feelings were always compounded by the guilt she felt when she overate.

Our first task was to help Val let go of her mistaken belief that she was a helpless victim of circumstances. She had to believe in her own power to change before change could be possible. When she was able to assume a more active stance, we moved to our "indirect" approach to weight loss. This involves finding better ways to satisfy needs currently met by overeating and overweight.

We started by exploring the costs and benefits of being overweight. To help with this analysis, we turned to Val's records of her weight-related feelings. Her diary indicated that she was embarrassed by her appearance when she met her son's teacher at school, and when she went to a family wedding. She was also acutely aware of her weight when she became overtired while doing housework, and while walking to the store. But her record also included feelings of relief when her husband made a snide remark about her tight-fitting pants, which she took as a sign that he wasn't going to approach her for sex. Other entries included:

> Saw an ad for a business program that was interesting. Doubted I'd get in. Then realized I couldn't even apply until I lose some weight.
>
> Was part of a mob scene at the "back-to-school" sale. Would have left, but I knew I was big enough to edge my way to the sale bins.
>
> Watched Don's buddies at the party coming on to any woman they saw standing alone. Knew they'd leave me alone. Funny—I was ashamed to be fat in front of the women at the wedding, but it was nice to be fat in front of the men.

These and other entries tipped us off to the ways that overweight helped Val. Val was embarrassed about her weight, but she also feared some of the consequences of weight loss. Her honesty about the benefits of being overweight enabled us to label these areas as necessary targets for change. Val had to confront her ambivalence about her extra weight in order to be ready to lose it. Specifically, she had to make the major change of learning to assert herself with words instead of weight.

Once Val resolved some of her fears about weight loss, we turned to the task of finding new ways to satisfy the emotional needs currently met by overeating. This time we used Val's eating diary to gather information about the circumstances, thoughts, and feelings that led to overeating.

Many of the major stresses in Val's life were related to her family. She felt inadequate in her dealings with her husband, her son, and her mother. These feelings of inadequacy regularly propelled her into the kitchen for a little psychic relief.

Like most people, Val had convinced herself that her circumstances could not be altered. We asked Val to reexamine her beliefs, and try to figure out where different choices could give her additional control. After exploring her conviction that her relationship with her husband was irremediably bad, she decided it couldn't hurt to ask him to join her for marriage counseling. We also had her examine her belief that only women should be caregivers. Eventually she worked up the courage to ask her brothers to help with their mother. And to bolster her self-esteem and lessen her boredom, she enrolled in a course at the local community college.

Then we turned to the circumstances that truly couldn't be changed. Her son was hyperactive, and other than making sure he took his medication, Val couldn't do much about his condition. Her mother was ailing and needed a great deal of care, and at least some of that care would fall on Val's shoulders.

At these times, Val could choose to suffer and feel miserable, or she could look for better ways to handle her feelings of helplessness and depression. With some brainstorming, Val was able to draw up a list of non-food related distractions to use when she was feeling down. She decided she could call a friend, indulge in a hot bath, or walk around the neighborhood when she felt the urge to eat. Armed with these resolutions, she set out to make changes that would make her less "hungry."

In general, we follow two simple rules for helping people gain more control over their lives:

1. *If a stressful situation can be changed, find a way to change it;*
2. *If a stressful situation can't be changed, find the best way to live with it.*

This may sound familiar; it's hardly original. The oldest source is the so-called "Serenity Prayer" which asks for "the strength to change what can be changed, the serenity to accept what can't be changed, and the wisdom to know the difference." This advice provides the foundation for designing a life in which stress is minimized, pleasurable activities are maximized, and overeating is therefore less necessary.

Generally, by the time we turn our attention directly to eating and exercise, some pounds have already disappeared, often without effort. As one woman said: "I had so many better things to do that I forgot about eating!"

IX

A Personal Touch

Once a woman is ready to lose weight, what can she do to be sure she'll succeed? We've been pondering this question for years, and every time we meet a woman who has lost weight, we try to find out what she did to reach her goal.

Most women start their stories by saying they woke up one morning and knew the time had come to be serious about weight loss. But the methods they used were far from uniform. Some started by giving up sweets entirely, eating only one meal a day, or eating only a few foods like cottage cheese and fruit. Others started by following a new diet recommended by a book, a magazine, or a friend. And still others joined weight control groups for structure and social support.

For most women, these approaches only worked for a week or two. Soon they found themselves deviating from their rigid weight-loss programs, and those who were determined to lose weight started to customize their weight loss plans to suit their own lifestyles. It is this flexibility that most often accounted for maintainable weight loss.

Acknowledging the fact that one program can't possibly suit

every woman's needs, we help women develop their own weight loss plans. We want to make sure that their successes or failures don't depend on their tolerance of liver or daily weigh-ins. Losing weight is difficult in the best of circumstances; there's no need to make the task harder by feeling forced to conform to unnecessary or offensive "rules."

Some women are disappointed when we don't give them a rigid, prepackaged plan. They have no faith in their own ability to make wise decisions, and they are accustomed to looking to "experts" for guidance and structure. We have to convince them that *they* are the only experts when it comes to their own lives. If they defer to the authority of others, they keep themselves in a passive and helpless role. When someone else makes the rules, the dieter is more likely to assert her authority by "cheating," even though she hurts herself by doing so. A woman can assure her own success only by taking active responsibility for designing and following her weight loss plan.

Once a woman is ready to design her own program, we supply the guidelines to help her create a plan that utilizes her strengths and helps her cope with her special challenges. While the details must vary, every personalized approach contains these essential elements:

1. An understanding of why most diets fail, in order to avoid these common pitfalls.
2. A plan for "phased" weight loss which allows time to make the necessary biological and psychological adjustments to a slimmer body.
3. An eating program that satisfies the body and the mind, thus combatting the tedium and stress generally associated with dieting, and paving the way for a lifetime of weight maintenance.

4. An exercise routine that makes it possible to lose and maintain weight while still being able to eat a satisfying amount of food.

5. A plan for managing binge eating that allows these eating crises to be opportunities to build new coping strategies.

In the following sections, we'll share our guidelines for designing personalized plans that substantially increase the likelihood of weight loss success.

GOOD INTENTIONS,
BAD RESULTS

Despite a history of dieting failures, the average woman in our study punishes herself by starting a diet at least five times a year. Rarely is she able to stick to it, and she typically regains the few pounds she loses in about twice the time it took to lose them.

Aside from the toll on health resulting from this "yo-yo" pattern,[14] women also pay the price of drastically lowered self-esteem. Once they abandon their diets, women always wonder "What's wrong with ME?" when they should be asking "What's wrong with this DIET?" Rather than condemn themselves, they should realize that no matter how bold a diet's promises, no matter how widely it's promoted, and no matter how many celebrities claim to have found new meaning in their lives by following it, *a diet's long-term effect is more likely to be weight GAIN than weight loss.*

Three biological factors account for the dismal failure rate of most diets. First, many fad diets are nutritionally imbalanced. All the essential nutrients can't be packed into diets containing fewer than approximately 1250 calories. A diet that includes too little protein leaves dieters constantly hungry. Diets low in carbohydrates can damage the liver, heart, and brain. And diets that don't include essential vitamins and minerals can lead to illnesses that can do irreversible harm.[15]

The body's only defense against the insult of long-term deprivation is to send signals in the form of intense food cravings, fatigue, and dizziness. At the price of self-injury, the dieter can try to outlast these discomforts. But the wise person will heed the signals and provide the fuel of food. Only the anorexic-in-training will be self-punishing enough to follow nutritionally imbalanced fad diets for more than a few weeks.

A second problem is even more vexing: the "starvation adjustment effect."[16] To understand it, we have to roll back several hundred thousand years. At that time, humans had little control over their food supply. Times of plenty were interspersed with times of famine. So human bodies developed a wonderful ability to store extra calories in the form of fat that could be converted into energy when food was scarce.[17]

This adaptive mechanism worked beautifully for women in the caves, who were more concerned with staying alive than with being able to feel their hip bones. But it is the bane of the modern woman's existence. Her body interprets skipped breakfasts and celery-stick lunches as signals that food is scarce. It responds by burning fewer calories and storing more as fat. The less she eats, the fewer calories her body burns. And each successive diet offers the body a little more training in how to slow its metabolic rate. So while a 1500 calorie diet may originally produce a rapid weight loss, eventually as few as 1000 calories a day may lead to weight gain![18]

As if the starvation adjustment isn't enough, researchers have found yet another villain that keeps weight loss at bay. A theoretical "set-point" appears to make it difficult for people to lose weight below a certain level.[19] Each person may have a biologically programmed minimum and maximum weight that can be surpassed only with great effort, if at all. It isn't clear whether the set-point is determined at birth or later in life, but one set of studies suggests that even a single sharp weight gain during adulthood can create a permanent disorder in the regulation of body weight.[20]

One of the pioneers of the set-point theory was Vermont researcher Ethan Sims.[21] Working with volunteer inmates in Vermont state prisons, he demonstrated that men given a long-term opportunity to eat twice as much as normal gained weight at very different rates. For example, if two started the experiment weighing 180 pounds, and both ate the same amount of food and had the same amount of exercise for the same number of days, one man might end the experiment weighing 195 and the other 225.

If there was a limit to weight gain, might weight loss be restricted too? This question was raised in another experiment conducted during World War II using conscientious objectors who volunteered to reduce their food intake by half.[22] Initially, there was a rapid weight loss, but eventually, most men's weight stabilized, and continued "starvation" did not lead to further weight loss. In addition, during the period of their weight loss, many of the men became clinically depressed, although nothing had changed but their food intake. As expected, when the experiment ended and the men could eat freely again, every one promptly regained most of the weight he'd lost.

These studies support the idea that each person has individually determined limits to weight gain and loss. To understand the implications for the dieter, let's imagine that a woman's body operates between high and low set points of 160 and 130 pounds. She might have to eat twice as much to move from 160 to 170 as she did to go from 150 to 160. By the same token, if she reduced her weight from 140 to 130 by following a 1500 calorie diet for six weeks, she might have to go down to 1100 calories for three months to lose the next 10 pounds. And 110 may elude her no matter what she does.

As if these biological obstacles aren't bad enough, the psychology of dieting also sentences many dieters to frustration and failure. This is partly due to their acceptance of one or more popular weight-loss fallacies. They are as follows:

Weight loss can be fast and permanent.

Everywhere, diet ads promise the loss of several pounds a day . . . effortlessly of course. Ignoring the fact that it's easier to consume calories than burn them, people naively try the "miracle" formulas that contain "secret fat-melting" compounds or "wonder diets" comprised of foods that "burn more calories than they contain."

Wishful thinking can lead a dieter to swallow many different kinds of bait, few of which will lead to anything but the loss of hope. While great expectations may help in losing a few pounds quickly, the weight invariably reappears . . . along with ten new wonder diets promising fast and permanent weight loss.

The best diets are the ones that are hardest to follow.

Too many dieters accept the premise that if it doesn't hurt, it will never work. So they choose diets for their torture value rather than their nutritive value. These diets are always started with great enthusiasm. A typical page from the determined dieter's food log might read:

Breakfast: a boiled egg, half a grapefruit, and one cup of coffee —black.

Lunch: half cup cottage cheese, small salad—no dressing.

The rest of the page is usually blank. It's too depressing to write "four jelly doughnuts" in the afternoon snack slot.

Deprivation diets don't work because they leave the dieter physiologically and psychologically starved for food. The greater the deprivation, the more irresistible "forbidden" foods become. Indeed everything in life seems to pale in importance when weighed against the pleasure of fresh baked bread or fudge brownies.

In addition, many popular diets require at least one bizarre ritual. One weight-control program used to forbid tomatoes after six P.M. and insisted that string beans had to be cut french style and no other way. Others allude to mixtures of chemicals in common foods that produce special effects. And some require secret-formula, foul-tasting liquids or pills of dubious composition. All of these gimmicks, calculated to lend the aura of "science," convince the dieter that she can't lose weight successfully without "professional" guidance and a multitude of rules.

Dieting is a temporary state of mind.

Most dieters console themselves by saying: "After I lose weight, I'll stop this punishment and go back to eating what I like." That thought is often the only thing that keeps them going. And who can blame them for not relishing the prospect of semi-starvation for the rest of their lives? That's a fate truly worse than fat!

But people who end diets by returning to old eating habits also quickly return to old weights. That's why so many people can lose weight, but so few can keep it off.

Every slip-up is a disaster.

Virtually every dieter strays from time to time. A few people are able to take these slip-ups in stride, without panic or self-reproach. They simply eat a little less at the next meal, or settle for a slightly slower rate of weight loss.

But the vast majority of dieters believe that the magic powers of their diet will only work if the diet is followed to the letter. To have any hope of succeeding, they think they must be perfect.

So when the inevitable slip-up occurs, it's seen as a personal disaster. And disaster is the best excuse for a good, serious, self-pitying binge.

These four dieting mistakes combine to form the infamous *diet-depression cycle.* Here's how it works:

- A woman waits until she's well over her goal weight. Then she panics, and decides she must lose weight immediately.
- Partly to punish herself for her excesses, and partly to help her get it over with as quickly as possible, she selects a trendy, very low-calorie diet.
- After following the diet for a short time, she begins to feel tired, irritable, and very much deprived. She starts to fantasize about everything she isn't allowed to eat, and soon finds herself obsessing about food.
- When other stresses build up, or when temptation is too close at hand, she gives in to her urge to "break" her diet. Telling herself that this is the last time she'll "cheat" until she reaches her goal, she decides to give in and really enjoy all her favorite foods for the rest of the day. She resolves to make a fresh start the following day.
- Feeling guilty about indulging herself the day before, she skips not only breakfast but also lunch.
- Soon those terrible feelings of deprivation take hold, and her resolve weakens yet again. This binge is even worse than the last, making it harder to fool herself about a better tomorrow.
- Still, she tries again. But the cycle just repeats itself: deprivation, overindulgence, guilt, increased deprivation, increased overindulgence, increased guilt . . . the cycle can continue for a lifetime.

Here's how one woman described her experience with the diet-depression cycle:

I've tried every diet there is, but I never have enough willpower to stay with it very long. I lose a few pounds, get depressed because I'm not losing fast enough, have a slip up, and take a giant slide.

When I diet, food is always on my mind. I try very hard not to overeat, but my stomach feels like an empty hole. So I keep going back for more food—some cereal, a piece of bread with peanut butter, then crackers or something else until I just stop noticing what I eat.

When I finally get to bed, I feel totally miserable, and make up my mind not to eat a thing the following day. By early afternoon, I always go back on my promise to myself. With each diet, I end up heavier than when I started. Of course that makes me more depressed. But I also get depressed when I'm not trying to lose weight, so I don't know where to turn.

On any given day, we estimate that one in every twelve American women is at some stage of this diet-depression cycle. It shouldn't come as a surprise that only a few will overcome the dual pressures of body and mind that doom most diets to failure. Does this mean that weight loss is an impossible dream? Obviously not. But successful, permanent weight loss requires the rejection of the dieting fallacies and the creation of a sensible, personalized weight loss plan.

PHASED WEIGHT LOSS

Most of the popular reducing programs promote rapid, large, and consistent weight loss. Promises of losing up to five pounds a week are not uncommon, and the implication is that goal weight will be achieved in an uninterrupted rush. Some organizations add the gimmick of a guarantee: if customers pay a huge fee up front, they'll be able to return for free service as long as they want—even though the service doesn't work.

We believe these claims are misleading, and the guarantees meaningless. Fast weight loss is seldom permanent, because the human body tends to resist rapid change. Weight is normally gained or lost at the rate of approximately eight-tenths of a pound per week.[23] When women lose two to four pounds a week during the first few weeks of a weight-control program, they're losing fluid, not fat. The rate will slow when the extra fluid is sloughed off; and the lost weight will return as soon as the fluid is replaced.[24]

To keep weight loss moving briskly, some programs recommend semi-starvation diets. But as every dieter knows, these diets are ineffective because they're inhumane. They create an inordinate hunger that must eventually be appeased. As a result, fat that's lost with "unnatural" speed usually finds its way back home just as quickly.[25]

Another problem with the goal of rapid weight loss is that it doesn't consider normal bodily changes. For example, most women have very *ir*regular patterns of weight loss due to factors such as premenstrual fluid retention. Set points and the starvation adjustment effect also take their toll. Many physiological realities lead women to hit plateaus at which they stop losing weight, despite continued dieting and exercise.

Weight-loss plateaus can also be related to emotional changes that accompany weight loss. As we've discussed, weight can provide protection from a variety of fears that intensify with weight loss. In addition, dieting women may be shocked when they don't recognize the "new" body reflected in their mirrors. They may feel that their new look requires a new personality to match, but they are either unwilling or unable to give up old patterns. This limits the appeal of further weight loss.

It doesn't make sense to advise a woman to keep cutting calories to get through the plateau. Instead, we ask her to take a breather from her weight-loss efforts by shifting to a weight-maintenance plan. This allows her body to adjust. It also gives her an opportunity to deal with any psychological issues that may be slowing her progress. Finally, she has time to incorporate her weight loss into a new body image, so that she can feel "at one" with her body.

In short, "phased weight loss" includes two guidelines:

1. *Plan gradual weight losses of one or two pounds per week;*
2. *Plan on taking a rest from losing weight after each 10 to 15 pound loss or whenever a plateau is reached.*

Gradual weight loss insures moderate caloric restriction and a moderate increase in physical activity. This avoids the hazards of risky diet and exercise programs. And the "rest stops" allow women to set short-term attainable goals, as well as allowing time to deal with any psychological issues that arise.

We ask our clients to expect their weight loss to follow a "step" pattern, in which they have time to adjust to each major change. We ask them to avoid the "slide" pattern, in which the only way they can stop themselves from hitting the skids is to reverse direction and start regaining weight. Weight loss may be faster using the slide approach, but it's more likely to be permanent with the step approach.

Even when they use the step approach, most women like to have an ultimate goal weight in mind. They find that having a goal makes it easier to "keep the faith" during difficult times, and it serves as a reminder that weight loss isn't a lifelong pursuit.

Choosing a goal weight is not as easy as it seems. For many years, doctors consulted standard charts to determine who needed to lose weight and how much they should lose. Recommendations were based on the assumption that overweight people were unhealthy. But recent research has shown that it's the amount of fat, not weight, that influences health.

To make matters more complicated, heredity plays a role. People with family histories of certain illnesses are more sensitive to the effects of weight gain than are those with healthier families. And personal habits also help determine how much fat is too much. For example, people who smoke or drink heavily have greater health risks at every weight than those who don't.

Because of these complexities, no single chart can replace a well-trained doctor's ability to gather the information needed to determine a person's ideal weight. Nevertheless, charts can offer a rough guideline for choosing a healthy weight.

The following chart was recently devised by the National Institute for the Aging. Different weights are suggested for different ages, because it's been found that gradual weight gain over the years is *not* necessarily harmful.[26] There's also a generous range within each category, to account for individual differences in bone structure and muscle mass. Finally, the chart doesn't differentiate between men and women, because the risks associated with each weight-by-height level are the same for all adults. We offer the following chart as the current "state of the art" for determining healthy goal weights.

Unfortunately, even doctors have a difficult time when they try to find reliable criteria for frame size.[28] So the woman at home must rely on very rough criteria. Because the methods used are crude and inaccurate, it's probably best to be conservative by using the *smallest* reasonable frame size.

It's important to remember that the weight ranges in this table are those within which the risk of contracting obesity-related diseases is *normal*. That means some people will get sick even at

WEIGHT RANGE
FOR MEN AND WOMEN BY AGE[27]

Height without shoes	Age				
	25	35	45	55	65
(ft–ins)	Weight without clothes				
4–10	84–111	92–119	99–127	107–135	115–142
4–11	87–115	95–123	103–131	111–139	119–147
5–0	90–119	98–127	106–135	114–143	123–152
5–1	93–123	101–131	110–140	118–148	127–157
5–2	96–127	105–136	113–144	122–153	131–163
5–3	99–131	108–140	117–149	126–158	135–168
5–4	102–135	112–145	121–151	130–163	140–173
5–5	106–140	114–149	125–159	134–168	144–179
5–6	109–144	119–154	129–164	138–174	148–184
5–7	112–148	122–159	133–169	143–179	153–190
5–8	116–153	126–163	137–174	147–184	158–196
5–9	119–157	130–168	141–179	151–190	162–201
5–10	122–162	134–173	145–184	156–195	167–207
5–11	126–167	137–178	149–190	160–201	172–213
6–0	129–171	141–183	153–195	165–207	177–219

the recommended weights depending on family history, past incidence of the disease, and the use of cigarettes, alcohol, and other drugs.

Also keep in mind that this chart refers to health, not beauty. There are no guarantees that a healthy weight is a "happy" weight. Physical attractiveness can't be measured statistically, it's a matter of individual taste. Some women in our survey consider fifty extra pounds to be "a little overweight" while others consider themselves "very much overweight" at five pounds above the lowest recommended healthy weight. We suggest choosing an initial goal weight within the healthy range, and then experimenting to find a weight that's also comfortable and attractive.

Once a comfortable goal weight is reached, it's useful to choose a "trigger weight" as a reminder that it's time to shed a few pounds. Trigger weights help women avoid sabotaging themselves by allowing too many pounds to accumulate before they take action. According to our research, women who maintain their goal weights use trigger weights of approximately five pounds above goal. In contrast, those who are 40 or more pounds overweight don't even think about losing weight until they're 15 to 20 pounds above goal.[29] By the time they decide to lose weight, the task seems too difficult.

Because it's much easier to find the motivation when there are only a few pounds to lose, we recommend using five pounds above goal weight as the trigger. This takes into account the normal weight fluctuations of three or four pounds that can occur in response to premenstrual fluid retention, temporary changes in activity, etc. By distinguishing between normal weight fluctuations and those that signal the need for determined effort, it will be easier to keep motivation high and weight stable.

A PERSONALIZED FOOD PLAN

Diet writers far away in Scarsdale or Beverly Hills don't know what Mrs. Smith in Topeka likes to eat. Whereas popular diets use a one-plan-fits-all philosophy, we advise every woman to do her own food planning. That's because every woman has different tastes, and she can be assured of daily eating pleasure only if she designs a food plan for herself.

The first step in planning a personal food plan is to determine how many calories can be consumed to achieve a healthy weight loss of one to two pounds per week, without causing hunger. Unfortunately, there's no simple way to identify the optimal caloric level. Some groups, like teenagers, pregnant and nursing women, and those who lead physically active lives, need more calories than others. And differences exist within groups because every body converts food to energy and fat at a different rate.[30]

Most women who are moderately overweight (e.g. 20 to 40 pounds above ideal weight), moderately active (e.g. planned aerobic activity like walking a few miles several times a week), and between 35 and 55 years of age will lose weight gradually on a plan in which they eat between 1,200 and 1,400 calories per day. But women with different degrees of overweight, who are more or less active, and who are older or younger might do better using different caloric levels.

For those who want to calculate an initial caloric level, the following formula, developed by registered dieticians Sachiko T. St. Jeor, Ph.D, R.D. and Jill Carlston, R.D. might be helpful. Three different numbers need to be plugged into the formula to estimate food energy needs to *maintain current weight:*

$$\left(\frac{}{A} + \frac{}{B} + \frac{}{C}\right) \times \frac{}{} \text{(current weight)} = \text{the number of}$$

calories that can be eaten daily without weight gain or loss.

    A. The first number is based on the degree of overweight:
        Choose *3* if 31 percent or more above ideal weight;
        Choose *4* if 11 to 30 percent above ideal weight;
        Choose *5* if 10 percent or less above ideal weight.
    B. The second number is based on the level of exercise:
        Choose *3* if exercise is infrequent or non-existent;

Choose 4 if exercise is light, e.g. 30 minutes or less, approximately three times a week;

Choose 5 if exercise is moderate, e.g. 30 minutes or more, four or more times a week.

C. The third number is based on age:

Choose 3 if 55 or older;

Choose 4 if 35 to 54;

Choose 5 if 34 or younger.

According to these guidelines, a woman who is: A. 60 percent above her ideal weight (3 calories), B. inactive (3 calories), C. 40 years old (4 calories) and who currently weighs 200 pounds should be able to eat approximately 2,000 calories per day without gaining weight:

$$[(3 + 3 + 4 = 10) \times 200 \text{ pounds} = 2{,}000 \text{ calories}]$$

If she went for a fast hour-long walk five days a week, this woman might be able to eat 2400 calories per day $[(3 + 5 + 4 = 12) \times 200 = 2400]$ and still maintain her present weight.

If this same woman wanted to *lose* weight, she would naturally need to lower her food intake. *Reducing calculated caloric intake by 500 calories per day often (but not always) results in a weekly weight loss of approximately one pound.* Thus a diet of 1900 calories per day could help this aerobically active woman lose approximately one pound per week.

At lower weights, the use of this formula must be adjusted. For example, a 30-year-old (5 calories), sedentary (3 calories) woman weighing 115 pounds (5 calories) would require approximately 1495 calories to maintain her weight $(5 + 3 + 5 = 13$ calories $\times 115)$. To lose weight, she might have to eat fewer than 1000 calories, and thereby risk the starvation adjustment effect and other hazards of severely restricted dieting. If she wanted to lose weight, she would be well advised to increase her physical activity rather than severely restrict her caloric intake. The more she exercises, the more she will be able to eat, while still losing weight.

These caloric levels are not magic, they're only averages. The actual numbers fluctuate because of many factors, only some of which we've mentioned. Therefore each woman will have to experiment to find the caloric level that works best for her. If she doesn't lose weight on her initial plan, she can decide to increase her activity and slightly decrease her food intake.

After deciding how much to eat, the next step is planning what to eat. In his authoritative guide, *Rating the Diets,* Theodore Berland offers many useful criteria for choosing a good food plan. He suggests asking questions like the following to determine which programs are best:

1. Was the program developed by a knowledgeable nutritionist or was it the creation of a movie star, a formerly fat person, or a well-meaning but uninformed popular writer?
2. Was the program tested and were the results reported in a respected professional journal, or are its benefits based solely on the author's self-reports?
3. Have all the principles upon which the program is based been made available for professional evaluation, or is the program based on "secrets" shielded from professional evaluation?
4. Has the food plan been shown to promote maintainable weight loss, or does it yield short-term losses at best?
5. Does the program provide all the essential nutrients, including adequate amounts of the necessary vitamins and minerals, or does it call for too few calories and/or an imbalanced assortment of foods?

To meet the body's nutritional requirements, the Select Committee on Nutrition and Human Needs of the United States Senate recommends food plans that are:

1. High in complex carbohydrates and fiber including fresh fruits, fresh vegetables, and whole grains;
2. Low in simple carbohydrates including sugar;
3. Low in high-cholesterol foods like red meat and whole-milk products, and high in foods with little cholesterol like fish, poultry, and skim-milk products;
4. Low in total fats, especially low in saturated fats;
5. Low in salt.

Two additional guidelines are also extremely important. A food plan must offer a variety of tastes, textures, and flavors to prevent it from becoming boring. Researchers have found that these qualities, rather than the quantity of food consumed, have the greatest impact on the feeling of being full and satisfied. Also, a physician's approval is recommended for everyone, and is crucial for anyone who suffers from nutrition-sensitive diseases like hypertension, diabetes, and hyperlipidemia, and anyone who has ever been advised not to lose weight.

It's also useful to limit consumption of prepackaged "diet" items. Although convenient, they are not without disadvantages. They cost more than foods without the "diet" label. Their caloric reduction is often obtained by heavy use of artificial ingredients, some of which may be unhealthy. They are rarely served to other family members, so the dieter (usually also the cook) may have to prepare at least two meals each evening. And their use does nothing to develop the skills needed to make wise choices in restaurants, or at home when the diet ends and maintenance begins.

Use of a "unit" food plan is one way to control the temptation to take one's calories in cookies and ice cream. (Good unit plans are included in *Getting Thin* by Gabe Mirkin, *The Nutritional Ages of Women* by Patricia Long, and *Jane Brody's Nutrition Book* by Jane Brody.) A unit plan provides the structure, but the dieter makes the specific choices. The plan provides lists of foods that have common nutritional characteristics, including similar caloric levels. For example, one slice of bread, 1/2 cup of hot cereal, or two 2 1/2 inch graham crackers have approximately equal calories and the same mix of nutrients. Once the dieter learns portion sizes, she'll have an easy time estimating the caloric level of all planned meals. And in addition to making meal planning easier, use of a unit plan is just as accurate as counting calories.[32]

Until the skill of estimating portion sizes is well developed, it's best to weigh or measure all servings carefully. A five-ounce piece of meat that's mistakenly believed to be three ounces leads to 150 extra calories. That mistake made daily means 1,500 extra calories a week and a one or two pound weight gain at the end of the month.

It's also important to keep accurate records of how much food is eaten. It's far too easy to "forget" that extra piece of toast or spoonful of jelly. And updating the written records *before* eating is the safest way to be sure they're accurate.

People who successfully lose weight don't stop at changing *what* they eat; they also change the *way* they eat. Here are a few examples of changes that help minimize overeating:

1. To Control the Frequency of Eating Urges
   a. Eat at about the same time each day. This helps the body develop a rhythm in which food is expected at selected times—not all the time.
   b. Keep the number of preplanned snacks to a minimum. This

reduces the number of daily exposures to food and makes it easier to divert attention away from eating.

c. Break the association between eating and other activities like watching TV or reading. This prevents "unconscious" eating, and increases enjoyment of food by allowing full concentration on eating.

d. Keep hard-to-resist foods out of the house, or keep them hidden if they must be in the house. The less often food is seen, the less frequent will be the urge to eat it.

2. TO INCREASE SATISFACTION WITH PORTION-CONTROLLED MEALS

a. Make portions seem larger by using smaller plates. Satiety is in the eye of the eater: satisfaction with portion size is strongly influenced by its apparent size.

b. Slow the pace of eating by cutting food into bite-size pieces, waiting two minutes before taking the first bit, swallowing completely before taking the next bite, and being the last person to begin eating each course. These changes allow greater pleasure from smaller amounts of food.

c. Decide how much to eat and eat only what was planned. Also, wait at least ten minutes after the main course before starting to eat dessert. Don't keep eating to feel full, because it takes about 20 minutes for the stomach to signal the brain that it has had enough.

3. MINIMIZE NIGHTTIME EATING

a. Curb late afternoon and evening fluid intake, particularly of caffeinated and alcoholic beverages. Sleeping through the night reduces the likelihood of middle-of-the-night snacks.

b. Plan alternatives to nighttime eating by keeping a book, knitting, stationery box or other diversion handy.

c. Plan nighttime snacks in advance, leaving them in containers. Most people choose high calorie foods when they go hunting in the kitchen late at night. Preplanned snacks reduce this risk.

d. Wait at least 10 minutes before getting out of bed and heading for the kitchen. Many people are able to fall asleep fairly quickly if they just stay in bed.

4. MINIMIZE EXPOSURE TO PROBLEM FOODS
   a. To reduce the likelihood of buying problem foods, shop from a list, with a friend, or after a full meal.
   b. Don't keep any food in the car or work area.
   c. Plan routes that avoid the need to drive or walk past shops offering food that is difficult to resist.
   d. Choose restaurants serving foods that are on the food plan, and order without looking at the menu. Be sure to ask that the food be prepared in the least-fattening manner.

A final word of caution is in order. Planning is a crucial part of a weight loss program. Women who plan too little gain too much. But those who *over* plan by choosing rigid programs are also in for a struggle. The mid-range food plan we recommend is structured, but preserves the freedom to maintain some eating enjoyment. It also draws upon the understanding that eating is as much a psychological as a physiological event. By building compassion into a food-plan, it's possible to take the agony out of losing weight.

THE ACTIVE SOLUTION

Contrary to popular belief, what a woman eats does *not* determine how much weight she'll lose. Instead, it's the *balance* between food intake and energy expenditure that results in weight gain or loss. Since eating too little can make it harder to lose weight, a plan for increased physical activity is an essential part of every successful weight-loss program.

The importance of exercise can't be overestimated. Here are some of the ways in which exercise makes weight loss easier:

1. It burns calories that might otherwise be stored as fat.
2. Whereas dieting often reduces metabolic rate, exercise can actually increase it.[33]
3. Moderate amounts of exercise actually reduce appetite.[34]
4. Moods and the ability to cope with stress greatly improve with moderate exercise.[35] Active people are less likely to feel fatigued, bored, tense, or depressed. And they generally find it easier to take stress in stride.
5. To lose weight through dieting alone, many women would have to cut their daily caloric intake to an extremely low level. This not only makes it harder to stick to a diet, but it usually slows metabolic rate, and retards weight loss.

Unfortunately, many people who have had lifelong battles with their weight feel that exercise is about as satisfying as a dinner of radishes and watercress. The common objections include lack of athletic ability, lack of time, and lack of a figure that looks good in a leotard or bathing suit.

There are also those who suffer from a "mental block" against exercise. They still harbor painful memories of being the last to be chosen for the softball team, or dangling helplessly at the bottom of the rope that everyone else could climb. For them, even the thought of exercise is associated with feelings of failure and humiliation.

Other people have good intentions, but lack the motivation to follow through. They buy the latest aerobics tape, then give up because they realize they'll never look like Jane Fonda. They spend $50 on running shoes, and then decide that it isn't really safe to be out on the streets alone. They sign up for tennis lessons, and then quit because the teacher is too impatient. They make plans to walk or jog with neighbors, but discover that it is much more fun to meet for cake and coffee.

It's easier to find reasons not to exercise than to find excuses for not losing weight. But if the excuses work, women deny themselves the safest, most effective way to burn extra calories, raise their metabolism, reduce their appetite, and improve their moods. Exercising may not come naturally, and it may not be easy, but for most people, it's the key to being thin.

Women who want to lose weight, and who are not now exercising, have a choice to make. They can decide that exercise is so unpleasant that they'd rather stay overweight. Or they can use their sweatsuits for something more than trips to the grocery store. Either choice makes more sense than wanting to lose a lot of weight solely by dieting; that decision is the sentence to a lifetime of frustration.

Women who decide to get more exercise should begin by choosing one or two forms that have the most appeal (or are the least unappealing). Walking, aerobics, use of an exercise bike or rowing machine, speed walking, jogging, and swimming are the most popular activities. Clearly these activities differ in convenience, expense, and sensitivity to weather. The advantages and disadvantages of each activity should be carefully considered before choosing an exercise plan.

Some people like to do the same activity every day, while others prefer a variety of activities. Some like to exercise alone, others prefer a partner or a group. Some would rather move at a leisurely pace for a longer period, while others prefer short-duration, higher-intensity activities. Some women may be unable to perform certain activities because of physical problems, expense, or inconvenience, but almost everyone can find at least one form of exercise that's acceptable.

It's important to choose activities that are likely to become—and remain—a part of a daily routine. Most women do best when they plan to exercise every day. Exercise then becomes a habit, rather than a daily decision. Activities do not have to be as rigid as swimming 25 laps or playing two sets of tennis. An after-dinner stroll or daily walk to the store may feel more relaxing and less like work.

The following suggestions can help establish a successful exercise program:

1. Plan to exercise at the same time each day so it becomes routine. Most people find they do best when they exercise in the early morning or late afternoon.
2. Develop "foul weather" alternatives. If walking is the chosen activity, it helps to locate an enclosed mall or several flights of indoor stairs that can be used when the weather is bad. Having an exercise bike or rowing machine at home is an even more convenient alternative.
3. Find ways to make exercise more interesting. A radio with headphones can be the jogger's best friend, and a TV set can prevent boredom while on a stationary bike. A variety of walking or running routes can also add stimulation and interest to an activity that might otherwise become dull.
4. Obtain medical approval before starting an exercise program. And consult a doctor about any signs of stress like dizziness, shortness of breath, rapid heartbeat, or acute pain that might signal the need for more moderate activity.
5. Finally, have alternative plans for coping with unexpected schedule changes. If it's necessary to go to work earlier than

usual, plan a 30 minute walk at lunch. On a business trip, try to allow time for an early morning walk through safe neighborhoods.

Remember that exercise is as important in preventing weight gain as it is in facilitating weight loss. If exercise ceases when goal weight is reached, the weight will not stay off for long. Fortunately, most people choose to stay active not just to keep their weight down, but because it feels so good!

BREAKING THE BINGE

I know I'm really hungry when a carrot or apple looks good. But when only sweets will do, the problem isn't hunger, and chances are that no amount of food will satisfy me. Still, once I give in to my desire to overeat, I can't stop it from becoming a full-blown binge.

Binge-eating plagues most overweight women. But the statement above was made by a woman who was at her goal weight. Two factors create this problem that troubles women of every size and shape. A full stomach never satisfies an emotional need, so psychologically motivated eating can be endless. And guilt about overeating only increases the negative feelings that lead a woman to overeat in the first place. Because overeating both pacifies and intensifies bad feelings, women can become "trapped" in an endless cycle of binge-eating and guilt.

There are two ways to view to binge-eating. *Perfectionists* believe that any deviation from a food plan is a catastrophe. Every time they give in to the urge to overeat, they punish themselves by feeling guilty, and then they either binge some more or purge themselves to emphasize their self-reproach. Not surprisingly, perfectionists are the architects of the diet–depression cycle. They set standards that no human being can meet, and then they berate themselves for failing to live up to their unrealistic expectations. Perfectionists can't help but suffer as a result of their inability to cope with predictable deviations from their ideals.

Realists, on the other hand, understand that occasional overeating is a fact of life. They see it as normal, and they try to minimize the damage of overeating by using what we call "binge-control reasoning." This involves analyzing the chain of events that leads to a binge, and learning how to break the chain at the earliest possible link. Preventing the binge from occurring is the best response. Interrupting it early is second best. Stopping before too much damage is done is still better than nothing. And at the very least, each binge should be analyzed after it's over to find ways to diminish future compulsive eating.

There are two keys to binge-control reasoning. The first is realizing that the *cause* of binge eating is feelings, never hunger, and the *cure* is dealing with the problem directly, not burying it with food. When a woman realizes that a binge is in the offing, answers to several questions can point her in the right direction: What am I really feeling? What can be changed, and what must be coped with? What besides eating will help me feel better?

The second element in binge-control reasoning is realizing that the desire to binge does not make binge-eating inevitable, and that even when a binge is in progress, it can be interrupted before it is complete. We believe that every binge involves four stages at which a variety of choices can be made.

The first stage is the *trigger.* A trigger is any feeling, thought, or action that stimulates the urge to overeat. As we've seen, common emotional triggers include feelings of boredom, anger, and frustration. Thought triggers include messages like "I'm the kind of person who can't resist chocolate," and "I was destined to be fat." Action triggers include skipping breakfast, or keeping a dish of candy in the living room "for company."

A woman has three choices when the urge to eat is triggered. She can take steps to *avoid* events that would trigger her urge to overeat in the future. This is her best move because it leads to long-term solutions that free her from having to resist temptation by preventing it from arising. For example, if boredom is a frequent trigger, a woman can put more variety in her daily routine and find some activities that give her a sense of accomplishment. If fatigue is a trigger for seeking a "sugar rush," she can eat an adequate breakfast every day to prevent mid-morning slump. If the "company candy" is irresistible, she can ask her husband to buy candy for guests the day they're expected to arrive. Or she can decide to serve her friends healthier snacks.

A second choice is to *escape* temptation with the least possible harm. Escape is usually a short-term action to control the urge, or appease it at the smallest possible cost. If a woman habitually tells herself that she's doomed to be fat because her parents were overweight, she can quickly replace the thought with the reminder that genes cause a predisposition to obesity, but they don't force anyone to be fat. If she skipped breakfast, she can respond to her hunger by having a healthy mid-morning snack. And if she is tempted by sweets in the house, she can freeze them. She can also do something enjoyable to give herself a "time-out."

The third alternative is the most familiar: giving in to the urge by indulging in favored foods. Because one bite is likely to lead to others, the binge eater enters the second stage of the cycle, *escalation*.

A woman again has three choices when a binge begins to escalate. She can *avoid* further compulsive eating by asking herself what she's trying to accomplish by eating, and dealing directly with the underlying problems instead of pacifying herself with food. For example, if she realizes that she's angry following an argument with her husband, she can talk with him about changes that can prevent similar arguments in the future. Or if she's bored, she can arrange to meet a friend. She can *escape* further eating by putting away the food and telling herself that she doesn't have to continue to eat just because she started. She can also eat fruit or vegetables instead of junk food. Or, once again, she can hit the skids by allowing the first spoonful of ice cream to "force" her to finish the quart.

If the cycle isn't interrupted, a binge is in full swing. But choices can still be made. Again it is possible to *avoid* catastrophe by seeing the binge as a sign of great stress and the need to find other ways to pacify emotions. A woman might decide to take a walk, write a letter, or call a friend. She can also *escape* with minimal damage by flushing the rest of the ice cream down the toilet or feeding the leftover roast beef to the dog. (We live by the motto that it's better to waste food than to wear it.)

As a last resort, she can eat until she's sick, feel overwhelmed with guilt, and resolve to atone with extreme self-denial (e.g. "I'm going to starve myself for the next three days"). This punishment will all but guarantee a bigger binge before the week is out.

Whether or not she feels guilty, a woman can decide *not* to punish herself, but rather to learn from the experience. This signals the start of the *recovery* stage, when the immediate crisis has passed. At this point, she can make plans to *avoid* the problem in the future. This might involve making life changes that can help improve her moods, or talking about her problems instead of stifling her feelings with food. Plans to *escape* future binges might include arranging a "hot line" with a friend who's also struggling with her weight. Many of our group members call each other for encouragement any time they feel they're heading for a binge.

The key to binge-control reasoning is to devise plans for interrupting the binge cycle at each of its stages, from the initial urge to the final remorseful bite. By accepting and understanding the desire to binge, it's possible to control it rather than to be controlled by it.

X

Two Heads
Can Be Better Than One

How can a husband help his wife lose weight? Should he join her, be a supportive bystander, or keep his distance?

The women in our study were clearly of two minds, in the classic tradition of "different strokes for different folks." A husband who gets involved might be praised or condemned; the same for the man who remains aloof. While it's clear that husbands are often blamed for making the weight-loss process harder than it has to be, wives are less clear about how husbands can do it right.

There is one area of absolute agreement: only a foolish husband tries to help his wife lose weight *before* she decides she wants to be thinner. Most wives are hurt when their husbands even *imply* that they're too fat: they feel attacked by the one person they counted on for support. As one woman explained:

> I constantly think about how fat I am, and what a failure I am for not being able to lose weight. My husband's bringing up the subject makes me feel worse. Not only is he telling me something I'm already painfully aware of, but he's reminding me that my appearance is more important to him than what's inside.

Naturally, the worse the relationship is, the more likely the wife is to take offense. But weight is such a sensitive issue that only women in the strongest, most secure relationships can take negative comments in stride. And even then, the husbands should choose their words carefully, and deliver the message with great tact.

Once a woman decides she wants to lose weight, some tangible help may be appreciated. Wives seem most appreciative when husbands share responsibility for feeding the family. Some men do the grocery shopping to spare their wives temptations that line each aisle. Others prepare family dinners so their wives can concentrate on preparing their own less caloric meals. And many take their children out for snacks instead of keeping goodies in the house. Every woman in our study appreciated help like this; their only complaint was that they weren't getting *more*.

Compliments about progress are always welcome unless they begin to sound like monitoring. As one woman put it:

> My husband is my "backbone" on dieting. But when he monitors every step I take, that's a little too much backbone! Encouraging me to stick to my diet all the time makes me defensive. When he remarks about the size of the portions I take, or notices when I don't have any "illegal" snacks, I feel he's intruding where he doesn't belong. My dieting is my business, and I wish he'd just leave me alone.

Other husbands go beyond practical help and verbal encouragement. They offer occasional gifts as incentives or rewards for weight loss. One woman was thrilled when her husband bought her sexy lingerie for Christmas: "I could fit into a few of the items, but most were too small. Each month, when I lost a little more weight, I could fit into something new. I would model it for my husband who was my one-man cheering section." But another wife was insulted when her husband gave her clothes that were three sizes too small. She felt unduly pressured to meet her husband's standards of thinness. As she tossed the clothes into her husband's arms, she told him to go find someone who'd fit them, because she was moving out.

When husbands "help" by criticizing their wives' diet efforts, perhaps by noting small lapses, they can expect a chilly response:

> My husband nags me even when I'm doing well on a diet and want just *one* sweet. That makes me so mad that I go out and binge on candy because I hate being told what to do. I've told him how I feel and he says he's just trying to help. I believe he's sincere, but with his help, I've gained 135 pounds in 13 years.

Obviously this husband isn't responsible for his wife's weight gain. He may have contributed to the problem by taking a parental role, but it's her choice to punish herself instead of redirecting him.

A husband who remains *un*involved with his wife's weight-loss efforts can appear a hero or a villain in her eyes. Some women interpret this as acceptance for who they are, not how they look. But others interpret a husband's inaction to mean: "He couldn't care less!"

About half of the women in our study claimed that if they were going to lose weight, they had to do it for themselves, not for anyone else. And these were the women who saw their husband's lack of pressure as the "highest form of respect a man could offer."

But an equal number of women were disappointed by their husbands' failure to help out. Many believed their husbands don't know what it's like to feel powerless against food. Others don't take the lack of support personally, but ascribe it to their husbands' general intolerance of "people who can't stand on their own two feet." But a significant number stated that their husbands simply "didn't give a damn." The most extreme reactions came from women in this latter group: those who chose to see sabotage where others might see only loving acceptance. This letter expresses the sentiments of more than a few women:

> Probably the nine most dangerous words he ever said to me were, "I will love you no matter what you weigh." Much as they were designed to pacify my anxieties about my weight, they became my license to overeat. His acceptance makes me too comfortable and too damned lazy about dieting. I sometimes wish he'd say "You lose or I leave." That would force my hand.

Although we respect each woman's right to choose the kind of help she wants from her husband, this sounds like an excuse to justify failure. Husbands, as we've seen, do sabotage their wives' weight-loss efforts in various ways, but acceptance isn't one of them. Not one woman told us she lost weight in response to her husband's pressure, unless losing weight was a first step in leaving him. We suspect that women who long for their husbands' disapproval would be none too happy if they got it.

In our clinical work with couples, we have had some opportunity to hear the husbands' views. The majority of men complain that it's boring to be around a person who spends so much time and energy worrying about what she eats and how she looks. Others say they just don't know what they're supposed to do—so they do nothing.

Confusion was certainly the primary reaction of the few well-meaning men who wrote in response to our survey. Frustrated about trying to help their wives, they asked for advice:

My wife is very pretty, except for her weight. I offered to take her on a big shopping spree when she loses weight, but nothing much happened. I tried bringing home diet foods, but that only made her angry. I'd like to learn how to be supportive without bringing up this painful subject all the time. I would gladly go out of my way to do whatever she wanted, but I'm at my wit's end as to how to help.

A husband has three choices when he doesn't know what to do. He can do nothing, he can use his imagination, or he can ask his wife what she would like. The men who want to help but don't know how usually end up offering the kind of help they'd want if they were trying to lose weight. Unfortunately, this is seldom the approach their wives would choose.

Men typically prefer action-oriented solutions to their problems, so that's what they offer their wives. They may buy exercise equipment and come up with "helpful hints" about what should and shouldn't be eaten. Or they'll offer "rewards" of money or clothes. They're trying to do what they'd want their wives to do if the situation were reversed.

However, women generally prefer emotional support and encouragement over practical tips and tangible rewards. They may be insulted by practical advice—they'd rather get that from the "experts." And gifts may be seen as bribery or coercion. When they're given what their husbands think they want, instead of what they themselves want, chances are they'll see the insult and ignore the good intent.

If all it takes is for a wife to tell her husband what she wants, why do so few bring up the subject? Sad to say, some women are reluctant to give up the excuse of uncooperative husbands. Others know what they want, but are afraid or ashamed to ask. But the majority simply don't know exactly what they mean when they say they want help. Some have trouble understanding why they compulsively overate in the first place. Some may want different kinds of help at different times. And some may have a vague idea of what they want, but not be able to express it.

To make life easier for both partners, wives should begin by examining their own feelings and deciding what behavior they would like from their husbands. The following questions may help to open up possibilities.

HOW CAN HE HELP?

1. What do you want your husband to do when he thinks you weigh too much?
    a. Say and do nothing.
    b. Ask me if I have been putting on weight lately.
    c. Tell me he thinks I could lose a few pounds.
    d. Other:_____

2. How do you want your husband to respond when you say that you think you've been gaining weight?
    a. Reassure me that I still look great.
    b. Ask if I want his help in losing weight.
    c. Tell me he agrees and that I should start a weight-loss program.
    d. Other:_____

3. Once you begin a weight loss program, what would you like your husband to do? (Choose as many alternatives as you want.)
    a. Do nothing. I want weight loss to be a solo effort.
    b. Exercise with me, at a pace that's comfortable for me.
    c. Eat the same foods I do, although in larger portions.

d. Take over some of the menu planning, food shopping, and/or food preparation.

e. Don't bring "forbidden" foods into the house.

f. Offer me incentives (such as gifts or nights out) for reaching specific interim weight loss goals.

g. Take the children out for treats that I can't have.

h. Surprise me with non-food gifts to keep my spirits up.

i. Other:_____

4. What do you want your husband do when he sees you making progress?

   a. Nothing: I want weight loss to be a solo effort and personal achievement.

   b. Let me know that he's impressed with my *efforts*.

   c. Tell me that he likes my *new appearance*.

   d. Other:_____

5. How would you like your husband to respond when he sees you lapse from your weight-loss plan?

   a. Do nothing: I know what I should do.

   b. Speak up only if he thinks things are getting out of control.

   c. Remind me every time so that small slip-ups don't become major catastrophes.

   d. Other:_____

Once a woman understands her own desires, she can ask her husband for help. Because this can be harder than it sounds, we'll point out a few of the potential problems.

Wives are often self-conscious about bringing up the subject, especially if they've spent years avoiding open discussion about their weight. They may feel defensive about admitting the need for help and risking possible refusal. Husbands may feel defensive if they interpret requests for change as implicit criticism, or if their past efforts to help didn't work.

Given the tension both partners may feel, it's easy for these discussions to get off on the wrong foot. Jabs like: "You've never been here for me when I need you!" "Why can't you be helpful for a change?" or "Sue says Jack has been a wonderful help to *her!*" will only make things worse.

Wives get better responses when they help their husbands listen undefensively, by making it clear that the husbands are not being blamed in any way. Asking for husbands' suggestions also increases the likelihood that they'll interpret the messages as requests, not accusations or demands. Vague, negative statements like the following won't do any good: "I'd like you to help me eat the right things." "You could support me when I'm doing well." "I'd like you to be interested but not involved." These statements express a goal, but without specifics about how to reach it. Trouble would result if a husband interpreted "right" to mean the foods *he* decides are proper, if "support" means giving presents a wife might resent, or "interested" means overseeing each morning's weigh-in. Being specific protects wives against the risk of misinterpretation.

Negative statements like "Don't tell me what to eat" are also useless, unless supplemented with positive requests. When all requests focus on what *not* to do, most husbands figure the best way to avoid mistakes is to do nothing at all.

Here's the advice we give our clients:

1. *Tell your husband you'd appreciate his help in your weight-loss attempt.* Make it clear that you are responsible for your own weight, but that there are things he can do to help. Say that you're making requests, not demands. And make enough requests so he can select the ones with which he's most comfortable.

2. *Keep your statements positive and specific,* so he doesn't have to read your mind. You can begin by showing him your responses to the quiz, and by clarifying items he doesn't understand. But then you'll have to go into greater detail.

Here are a few examples:

> Every time you see me reach for seconds, please ask me if I'm eating because I'm hungry or because there's nothing else to do. But only ask once: from then on it's up to me.

> I know you like to eat candy in the movies and you know I can't stop eating it once I start. When we go to the show, please buy only licorice, because it's the only kind of candy you like that I won't even taste.

3. *Solicit your husband's views.* Ask him how he feels about your decision to lose weight. Does he support it? Does he have any fears about changes that might occur as a result of the weight loss? Does he wonder if you will expect him to lose weight, give up drinking, or make other major changes? Have there been problems associated with past weight loss attempts (such as irritability, diminished social life, etc.) that make him reluctant to support your efforts?

4. *If he accepts your decision to lose weight, find out how he feels about the specific requests you've made.* Are there any that he finds objectionable or particularly difficult? Are there any that he doesn't understand? Is there anything you can do to make it easier for him to support your efforts?

Not all husbands will feel comfortable with this kind of conversation. Some men shy away from "feeling talk," while others try to avoid any kind of talk at all. Still, it doesn't hurt to try. The worst that will happen is that a wife will realize that she has to do it on her own. But with luck, she'll discover that her husband is happy to lend a hand, once he knows what he can do to help.

Epilogue:
Staying Hopeful

Like others who have tried to discover the secret of permanent weight loss, we've fluctuated between cautious optimism and reluctant pessimism. Currently, we're feeling hopeful. We don't believe that weight loss is necessarily easy, nor are we convinced that it's always possible. But by uncovering the common obstacles to successful weight loss, we've been able to solve at least some of the mystery of failed weight-loss attempts.

Several themes keep turning up in our work with overweight women:

1. *Overeating is usually a reasonable response to a woman's life.* It's an attempt to cope with her feelings and fears as best she can. Until she learns better ways of handling these stresses, weight loss attempts are likely to be futile.
2. *Overweight is not without its benefits.* Until a woman comes to terms with the advantages of being fat, she'll have a hard time feeling comfortable with being thin.
3. *Nobody is a helpless victim.* No matter what a person's circumstances, there is some choice as to how to react. Every woman has the power to create positive change.

4. *Weight loss does not have to be a constant test of self-control.*
Most women make their task harder than necessary: it does
not make sense to bake brownies when feeling depressed or
anxious, and then try to eat just one. It's important to
understand the different choice points in the overeating
cycle, and to learn how to interrupt the cycle early, before
emotions overrule reason.

5. *Self-designed weight-control programs work better than prepackaged plans.* Every woman is different, and no one plan can
meet all women's needs. While it takes more work to
develop a personalized plan, the results are worth the effort.

6. *Too many women spend too much time thinking about food and
weight.* This preoccupation distracts them from more re-
warding concerns. Directing attention away from food and
fat can be the best way to conquer a weight problem.

Barbara's story illustrates this last principle very well. After
focusing for years on food and weight, she decided to give up.
Since nothing she tried worked for more than a few weeks, all
the time and effort seemed futile. So she began to pay attention
to other things like work, friendships, and having fun. She also
decided that if she couldn't be thin, she could at least be healthy,
so she started an exercise routine. (The first week, she had to work
up to running a quarter of a mile each day, but she gave herself
credit for putting on her sweatsuit and getting out of the house!)

Barbara gave away her scale, so she had no idea what was
happening to her weight. But in time—a year, perhaps two—
the extra weight disappeared. She was oblivious to the weight
loss, and continued to buy clothes that were several sizes too
large. Even when she finally acknowledged that she was thin, she
saved all her "fat" clothes because she was sure she'd need them
again. Since she had done nothing deliberately to lose the weight,
she was sure that her eating problems, and extra weight, could
reappear at any time.

It's been almost eight years since Barbara has had any problem with her weight. But the tent dresses have been given to pregnant friends, and the other large clothes donated to charity, because she no longer fears weight gain. This newfound confidence is the direct result of some of the lessons we've learned. For those who worry about regaining lost weight, these principles may be useful:

1. *Every slip-up should be treated as an opportunity to evaluate the need for change.* For example, the desire to binge-eat is not a disaster, or an omen of returning "illness." Occasional urges to overeat are normal, and frequent urges should serve as cues to take problem-solving action.
2. *It's important to take action as soon as the need for action is clear.* Problems rarely go away by themselves: they're more likely to grow with the passage of time. The use of five-pound "trigger weights" can prevent small weight gains from becoming large ones.
3. *Weight gain or loss is the result of the balance between food intake and activity.* Most women decide to starve themselves when they want to shed a few pounds. A better approach would be a moderate increase in activity coupled with a modest decrease in caloric intake. Exercise is far superior to dieting as a means of diminishing nervous tension, combatting depression, and decreasing appetite.
4. *Weight control is a personal issue, but helpful social support always makes the task easier.* Whatever kind of help a woman wants, she'll have an easier time managing her weight if she asks for and receives support for her efforts.

Even when their families are helpful, many women enjoy the additional support provided by a group. Our weight-loss groups have stimulated women to explore their feelings about food and fat, and find new ways to approach these sensitive issues. We've recently realized, however, that to give these groups the label "weight loss" is to require women to choose that goal before carefully considering implications and alternatives. Therefore, we've changed the name of our program to Eating Awareness Group.™

Our groups begin with several weeks of discussion about the personal meaning of overweight. Once the benefits of being fat have been identified, our next step is to help members find alternative ways to achieve the same results at a lower personal cost. Even with these new skills in place, some women decide they'd rather be fat than thin; our challenge is to help them develop a positive self-image that isn't keyed to weight. For those women who choose to lose weight, we focus on helping them understand how they use food to cope with troubling emotions.

Being in a group is particularly useful for finding ways to break the food-mood connection. Most members feel that eating is not only a logical response to situations in their own lives, it's the only response. But when they listen to other women's accounts, they can see ways in which fatalistic or simplistic thinking leads to faulty conclusions. As they help others develop more constructive thinking, they learn to apply the same principles to themselves. It's then much easier to create personalized action plans with a greater chance of success.

Once each woman knows what she wants to accomplish, the group supplements the help received at home, or provides support if it's not available elsewhere. The value of talking with women who have similar problems is tremendous. Members not only help each other with new coping skills, they also provide the support that's needed to transform these skills into habits.

Readers who cannot join our Eating Awareness program might be interested in our personalized Eating Awareness Inventory, computer analyzed to yield a printout with detailed information about whether a woman should lose weight; how she can change the way she thinks, feels, and acts in order to lose weight more easily; how she can enlist from others the kind of help she wants; and suggestions for a food and exercise plan tailored to her individual needs. Send a self-addressed envelope to Compuscore, Box 7035, Ann Arbor, Michigan, 48107, and the Inventory will be mailed to you.

Whether a woman joins a group or goes it alone, discovering the personal meanings of food and fat can give her a new lease on life. By identifying her unstated assumptions about her body image, she can be free to choose the weight at which she'll be most comfortable. By discarding the belief that she is doomed to be a victim, she can assert more control over her life. And by taking a critical look at her closest relationships, she can work toward improving any patterns that have eroded her self-esteem.

How will these changes affect her weight? Only the woman herself can make this decision. She may choose to accept herself as she is, or she may increase her determination to lose weight. Aided by greater understanding and self-acceptance, she'll be far more likely to meet her goal, whatever it may be.

Notes

1 Stuart, R. B., & Jacobson, B., "Sex Differences in Obesity," in: *Gender and disordered behavior* edited by E. S. Gomberg & V. Franks (New York Brunner/Mazel, 1979).

2 Boynton, S., *Chocolate, The Consuming Passion* (New York: Workman Publishing, 1982), p. 57.

3 Burum, Linda., *Brownies* (New York: Scribner's, 1984).

4 *Peppridge Farm Gift Catalogue*, (1986), p. 34.

5 Blumstein, P. and Schwartz, P., *American Couples* (New York: William Morrow, 1983), p. 202.

6 McGill, M., *The McGill Report on Male Intimacy* (New York: Holt, Rinehart, and Winston, 1985), p. 64.

7 Wheelis, Allen, *How People Change* (New York: Harper & Row, 1973), p. 115.

8 Ibid., p. 31.

9 Huenemann, T. L., L. R. Shapiro, M.C. Hampton, and B. W. Mitchell, "A longitudinal study of gross body composition and body conformation and their association with food and activity in a teen-age population," *American Journal of Clinical Nutrition* (1966) 18:325–38.

10 Allon, N., "The stigma of overweight in everyday life," in *Psycho-*

logical aspects of obesity: A handbook, edited by B.B. Wolman (New York: Van Nostrand Reinhold & Co, 1982) pp. 130–74.

[11] Roe, D. A., and K. R. Eickwort "Relationships between obesity and associated health factors with unemployment among low income women." *Journal of the American Medical Women's Association* (1976) 31:193–204.

[12] "Fear of fat: The medical evidence," *Consumer Reports* (August, 1985): 455–57.

[13] Wheelis, *op.cit.,* 16–17.

[14] U.S. Public Health Service. *Obesity and health* (Washington, D.C.: U.S. Government Printing Office, n.d.).

[15] Mayer, J., "Weight control and 'diets:' Facts and fads," in S. Barrett, and G. Knight *The Health Robbers: How to Protect Your Money and Your Life,* edited by S. Barrett and G. Knight (Philadelphia: George F. Stickley Co. Publishers, 1976), pp. 50–51. Sours, H. E., V. P. Frattali, D. Brand, R. A. Feldman, A. L. Forbes, R. C. Swanson, and A. L. Paris, "Sudden death associated with very low calorie weight reduction regimens," *The American Journal of Clinical Nutrition* 34 (1981) 453461; Wadden, T. A., A. J. Stunkard, and K. D. Brownell, "Very low calorie diets: Their efficacy, safety, and future," *Annals of Internal Medicine* (1983) 99:675–84.

[16] Apfelbaum, M., "Adaptation to changes in caloric intake," *Progress in Food and Nutritional Science* (1978) 2:543559.

[17] Beller, A. S., *Fat and thin: A natural history of obesity* (New York: Farrar, Straus, & Giroux, 1977).

[18] Blondheim, S. H., N. A. Kaufman, and M. Stein, "Comparison of fasting and 800–1000 calorie diet in obesity," *Lancet* (1965) 1:250–52.

[19] Keesey, R. E., and T. L. Powley, "Regulation of body weight," *Annual Review of Psychology* (1986) 37:1-9-133; Nisbett, R. E., "Hunger, obesity, and the ventromedial thalamus," *Psychological Review* (1972) 79:433–53.

[20] Faust, I.M., "Role of the fat cell in energy balance and physiology" in *Eating and its disorders,* edited by A. J. Stunkard and E Stellar (New York: Raven Press, 1984), pp. 97–107.

21 Sims, E. A. H., "Studies in human hyperphagia," in *Treatment and Management of Obesity,* edited by G. Bray and J. Bethune (New York: Harper & Row, 1974).

22 Keys, A., HJ. Brozek, A. Henschel, O. Mickelson, and H. L. Taylor, *The Biology of Human Starvation* (Minneapolis: University of Minnesota Press, 1950).

23 Bortz, W. M., "Predictability of weight loss," *Journal of the American Medical Association* (1968) 204:99–105.

24 Stuart, R. B., J. Jensen, K. Guire, "Weight loss over time: Concomitants and consequences of decreasing rate" *Journal of the American Dietetic Association* (1979) 75:258–61.

25 Stuart, R. B., C. Mitchell, and J. Jensen, "Planning and predicting the results of obesity therapy," in *Medical psychology: A new perspective,* edited by L. A. Bradley and C. K. Prokop (Philadelphia: W. B. Saunders, 1980), pp. 321–53.

26 Andres, R., D. Elahi, J. D. Tobin, D. C. Muller, and L. Brant, "Impact of age on weight goals," *Annals of Internal Medicine* (1985) 103, pt. 2:1030–33

27 Ibid. Reprinted with the permission of the authors.

28 Simopoulos, A. P., "Obesity and body weight standards." *Annual Review of Public Health* (1986) 7:481–92.

29 Stuart, R.B, Guire, K. "Some correlates of the maintenance of weight lost through behavior modification." *International Journal of Obesity* (1979) 3:87–96.

30 Auckland, J. N., E. Morrison, and C. Hunt, "Slimming experience among college students: Variability in metabolic rate between and within individuals and its relevance to 'success' in slimming," *Journal of Research on School Health* (1984) 2:58–61.

31 Garrow, J. S., M. L. Durrant, S. Mann, S. F. Stalley, and P. M. Warwick, "Factors determining weight loss in obese patients in a metabolic ward," *International Journal of Obesity* (1978) 2:441–47; Stokholm, K. H., and M. S. Hansen, "Lowering of serum T3 during a conventional slimming routine," *International Journal of Obesity* (1983) 7:195–99.

32 Wing, R., R., M. P. Nowalk, L. H. Epstein, and R. Koeske,

"Calorie-counting compared to exchange system diets in the treatment of overweight patients with Type II diabetes," *Addictive Behaviors* (1986) 11:163–68.

33 Donahoe, C. P., D. H. Lin, D.S. Kirschenbaum, and R. E. Keesey, "Metabolic consequences of dieting and exercise in the treatment of obesity, *Journal of Consulting and Clinical Psychology* (1984) 52:-827–36.

34 Stuart, R. B., "Exercise prescription in weight management: Advantages, techniques, and obstacles," *Obesity and Bariatric Medicine* (1975) 40:16–24.

35 Roth, D.L., and D. S. Holmes, "Influence of physical fitness in determining the impact of stressful life events on physical and psychologic health," *Psychosomatic Medicine* (1985) 47:164–73.

Index

abused wives:
  anger of, 60
  eating as consolation, 46–47
  extramarital affairs of, 53
  self-liberation by, 103
  toleration of abuse, 47–48
  weight loss as cause of abuse, 72, 82
Act Thin, Stay Thin (Stuart), 17
addiction to food, 41, 46
agoraphobia, 63
alcoholism:
  of husbands, 46, 75
  treatment for, 18–19
anger suppressed with overeating,
  60–61
anorexia, 93, 115
"attractive" weight levels, 146–47

behavioral self-management, 15
behavior modification programs, 16
Berland, Theodore, 150
binge-control reasoning, 159–62
binge-eating:
  cycle of, 93–94, 158

dieters' attitudes toward, 158–59
  escalation stage, 160–61
  full swing stage, 161
  recovery stage, 161
  trigger stage, 159–60
birth control, 59
bored eaters, 31–33, 128
Brody, Jane, 152
bulimia, 93

caloric intake formula, 148–50
Carlston, Jill, 148
casual eaters, 127–28
chocolate as substitute for love, 34–35
coping eaters, 128–29
courtship, 24–25

depression:
  diet-depression cycle, 141–42, 159
  of housewives, 28–30
  marriage as solution to, 23
  weight loss as cause of, 138
diabetes, 98, 124

diet-depression cycle, 141–42, 159
"diet" foods, 151
diets:
  bizarre rituals, 140
  deprivation diets, 139–40, 143
  nutritional imbalance in, 136–37
  obsession with dieting, 93–94
  rapid weight loss through, 142–43
  "set point" theory of weight and,
    137–39
  sexuality, effect on, 110–11
  slip-ups, 140–41
  starvation adjustment effect and,
    137
  temporary nature of, 140
  weight-loss fallacies, 139–41
  yo-yo pattern of dieting, 136
direct approach to weight loss, 21,
    126–27
diverticulitis, 117

Eating Awareness Group, 176
Eating Awareness Inventory, 176–77
eating diary, 129, 131
eating habits, changing of, 152–54
"eating orgasms," 35
excuses for overeating, 87–88
exercise, 154–55, 175
  daily routines, 157
  medical approval, 157
  motivation problems, 155–56
  negative attitudes toward, 155
  program development, 156–58
  weight loss and, 155
  for weight maintenance, 158
exercise specialists, 15
extramarital affairs:
  of husbands, 76–77
  husband's fears regarding wife's
    possible affairs, 77–79, 81
  weight loss as cause of, 53–56, 79

fat distribution in women, 115–16
food plan, 21
  benefits of, 154
  caloric level, determination of,
    148–50
  "diet" foods, avoidance of, 151
  foods included in, 150–51
  medical approval, 151
  personalization of, 147–48
  portion sizes, 152, 153
  record-keeping, 152
  unit plans, 152
  variety in, 151
frame size, 145
friendship deterioration due to weight
  loss, 105, 106

genetic predisposition for obesity, 88
Getting Thin (Mirkin), 152
goal-weight selection, 144–47

health problems of obesity, 98
heart disease, 98
housewives:
  adult companionship, lack of, 30–31
  boredom of, 31–33, 128
  depression of, 28–30
  fatigue of, 31
  fattening nature of the work, 27–28
  overeating as release from stress, 33
  past employment, 30
How People Change (Wheelis), 89
husbands:
  alcoholics, 46, 75
  changes related to weight loss,
    inability to adapt to, 106–9
  extramarital affairs of, 76–77
  insecurity of, 77–79
  intimacy, attitudes toward, 39–40
  jealousy due to weight loss, 109–10